Biomechanics and energetics
of muscular exercise

Biomechanics and energetics of muscular exercise

BY

RODOLFO   MARGARIA

CLARENDON PRESS · OXFORD
1976

Oxford University Press, Walton Street, Oxford, OX2 6DP

OXFORD LONDON GLASGOW NEW YORK
TORONTO MELBOURNE WELLINGTON CAPE TOWN
IBADAN NAIROBI DAR ES SALAAM LUSAKA ADDIS ABABA
KUALA LUMPUR SINGAPORE JAKARTA HONG KONG TOKYO
DELHI BOMBAY CALCUTTA MADRAS KARACHI

ISBN   0   19   857397   9

© Oxford University Press 1976

Typeset in Northern Ireland at The Universities Press (Belfast) Ltd.

Printed in Great Britain at the University Press, Oxford
by Vivian Ridler, Printer to the University

Preface

I FIND the physiology of muscular exercise one of the most stimulating branches of biology and the one of the widest interest, not only because the movement of the body is one of the most characteristic activities of all animals, but also because it results in the greatest energy transformations that the body undergoes. For example, oxygen consumption, which may be considered as an index of the intensity of chemical and energetic metabolism, increases in man some 15 to 20 times from the value at rest under conditions of maximal aerobic activity; in maximal exercise of short duration the rate of anaerobic transformation increases to an even greater extent.

Muscular exercise may therefore be regarded as an 'amplifier' of the chemical and energetic metabolism. The study of the chemical transformations that take place in the body is easier and more susceptible to a quantitative treatment under conditions of muscular activity; it is as though we were looking at these functions with a magnifying lens. During muscular exercise the activity of the heart and the circulation in general increases, as does respiration, the activity of the nervous system, the digestive and secretory functions, etc. Students of all branches of physiology therefore need a sound knowledge of the physiology of exercise. The subject should be of interest not only to scientists, but also to all educated people because of its practical applications.

For example, certain biochemicals may, because of metabolic errors, accumulate in the body which in high concentration may be harmful and have a toxic effect. When the rate of metabolism of the body as a whole is increased by exercise, the catabolism of these substances is also increased, and they no longer reach a harmful concentration. A more direct application of the physiology of muscular exercise is the measurement of the maximum muscular power of an individual. I think this is a more important characteristic than the commonly collected anthropometric data such as height, weight, perimeter of the chest, etc., for it enables a prediction of potential performance, and gives more direct information on the functional capability of the individual. It is easily measured by the method described in Chapter 1. Unfortunately, this idea has not yet found practical application, even in ergonomics, a subject that is of interest because of its applications in work and production. Nor has it been applied in sport and recreation.

Every individual, and the organization to which he belongs, should know his maximum muscular power. An athlete should also be well informed about muscle physiology, the biomechanics of movement, and muscle energetics, in order to be able to attain maximum efficiency in the exercise that he is performing.

A knowledge of the aerobic and anaerobic maximum muscular power of an individual is also important in preventive medicine. Measurement of maximal muscular power, particularly the aerobic maximal muscular power, of a patient is an integrative test, as there are converging on it the contributions of other systems—besides the nervous and the muscular ones—such as the cardiocirculatory and the respiratory systems. Therefore a low value may be an index of a depressed function of one of these systems. The same test may be applied to study the effect of a therapeutic measure on the organism: its intervention may be chemical, pharmacological, physiotherapeutic, or psychological. A practising physician is obviously bound to specify the amount of a pharmacological prescription: he should also be able to prescribe exactly the quantity and intensity of muscular exercise that he suggests to his patients. The lack of an exact quantitative prescription may lead to the same inconveniences and dangers of a wrong dosage of a drug.

The contents and the style of this book are very personal and relate mainly to the research that I have carried out in the last ten years in the Institute of Human Physiology of the Medical School of the University of Milan. The book deals with the aspects of muscle physiology and exercise that I think are the most interesting and important, and that had awakened the passion and the interest of all our group for a long time. I hope that this book, which is intended to cover the fundamentals of the physiology of exercise, will stimulate research, not only by physiologists, but also by physicians interested in occupational medicine, ergonomics, and sports, and by physical educators, who would thereby learn to rely more on basic physiological concepts in their daily work. At present numerous prejudices, wrong notions, and empirical concepts hinder a proper understanding of muscular performance and these are difficult to eradicate.

I should like to thank very warmly my friends from overseas who are in a way the patrons of this book: particularly Professor J. Milic-Emili of Montreal, who started his brilliant university career in my Institute in Milan and to whom I am very deeply indebted culturally and personally; my good friend from the Fatigue Laboratory, D. B. Dill of Boulder City (University of Nevada); and many others, including Professors Devenport and Faulkner of Ann Arbor, Ricci of Amherst, Taylor of Cambridge, Ferguson of Montreal, Thoden of Ottawa, Macklem of Montreal, Landry of Quebec, Shephard of Toronto, Clements and McIllroy of San Francisco, and Josenhans of Halifax. My thanks are due also to all my collaborators of the Institute and lastly to the staff of the Oxford University Press, who did a superb job in brushing up my English.

Milan, 1975   R.M.

Contents

1. ENERGY SOURCES IN MUSCULAR EXERCISES   1
Introduction, 1. A few historical notes, 1. The fundamental chemical reactions in muscle, 6. The energy from oxidations, 9. The energy equivalent of the glycolytic process, 9. The energy equivalent of lactic acid formation from glycogen, 12. The calculation of the maximum aerobic power from blood lactic acid, 17. Lactic acid in submaximal exercise, 18. Capacity and power of the glycolytic mechanism, 20. Capacity and power of the alactic mechanism, 21. Anaerobic recovery, 27. Possible variations of the capacity and power of the alactic mechanism, 29. The oxygen debt, 29. The measurement of the oxygen debt, 30. The alactic oxygen debt, 31. Net and gross alactic oxygen debt. The kinetics of the alactic oxygen debt payment, 32. Summary concerning the exergonic processes in muscle, 33. The measurement of the maximum muscular power, 35. Maximum anaerobic power, 35. The maximum aerobic power, 37. A simple relationship between maximum aerobic power and performance in running, 43. Intermittent strenuous exercise, 46. Delayed production of lactic acid, 48. The course of the contraction and payment of the oxygen debt in supramaximal exercise, 50. A hydraulic model of the energetic processes in muscle, 53. The efficiency of the processes involved in energy transformation, 55. Energy equivalent of phosphagen cleavage and lactic acid formation, 56.

2. SOME FUNDAMENTAL CARDIORESPIRATORY FUNCTIONAL CHANGES MET IN EXERCISE AND OTHER CONDITIONS   59

3. BIOMECHANICS OF HUMAN LOCOMOTION   67
Introduction, 66. The energy cost of walking at a constant speed, 66. Energy cost of running, 73. The mechanical efficiency of walking and running, 74. Positive and negative work, 77. The force–velocity diagram of the active muscle, 78. Energy transformations in positive- and negative-work performance, 80. The measurement of mechanical work, 80. External and internal work, 83. Potential and kinetic energy changes in walking, 84. A mechanical model of walking, 85. High-speed walking, 87. The mechanics of running, 89. The phases of the

potential and kinetic energy changes in walking and running, 92. A mechanical model of running, 94. The mechanical efficiency of running, 96. External and internal resistances in walking and running, 100. External frictional resistances, 101. 'Wasted' mechanical work in locomotion, 103. The wheel model of human locomotion, 105. Measurement of maximum muscle power during running, 108. The rate of positive and negative work in walking, 111. The effect of a steady pull on the energy expenditure in walking, 113. The utilization of the elastic energy in muscular exercise, 115. Utilization of the elastic energy in the isolated muscle. Force–length diagrams, 120. Walking and running as oscillatory phenomena, 123. The influence of gravity on human locomotion, 126. Walking and running on the moon, 128. Progressing by jumps in sub-gravity, 130. Energy cost of locomotion on the moon, 132. Sprinting in sub-gravity, 133. The effect of gravity on jumping 134.

REFERENCES   140

INDEX   145

1 Energy sources in muscular exercise

Introduction

A MUSCLE is a machine that generates mechanical energy (it performs work) at the expense of chemical energy by transforming substances that have either been previously formed in the muscle, or that reach it through the circulation. It is, therefore, an engine.

The most significant characteristics of an engine are the mechanical energy produced, i.e. the work that it can perform, and the energy required to make it function. In physiology, the measurement of the mechanical work performed is relatively easy; instruments called 'ergometers', such as the treadmill, the bicycle ergometer, etc., have been constructed for this specific purpose and are widely employed.

Measurement of the energy expended in operating a man-made motor is usually simple; if it is an electric motor, the voltage and the intensity of the current feeding the motor must be known; if it is a combustion engine, the amount of fuel that is consumed can be measured; and so on. In the case of muscles, the measurement is much more complex because, among other things, there are various sources of energy that directly or indirectly are utilized in activity, and the measurement of each of them may be very elaborate. An accurate energy balance can be accomplished only after a detailed quantitative analysis has been made of each of the sources of energy, and when it is known at what time, or stage, they intervene, as related to the production of mechanical work.

A few historical notes

It has been known for a long time that the amount of energy transformed in muscular exercise is proportional to the oxygen consumption; the ultimate source of energy must therefore in all cases be combustion. Muscle is not, however, a combustion engine, and the chemical reactions directly involved in the immediate supply of energy for the production of mechanical work are not oxidative.

In fact as is well known, muscle can perform a long series of contractions in the absence of oxygen, and the mechanical characteristics of the contraction, as well as the heat production, the electrophysiological processes, etc. are exactly the same whether oxygen is available or not: the only difference is that in the absence of oxygen the capacity for performing prolonged work is very limited.

The fundamental chemical reactions providing energy for accomplishment of mechanical work are evidently *anaerobic*. In the 1920s this reaction was thought to be the *formation of lactic acid from glycogen* (glycolysis). This theory substantially derived from a long and careful analysis by A. V. Hill of heat production in the isolated muscle, as related to the mechanical work performed, and from the analysis performed by O. Meyerhof of the chemical changes taking place in muscle. These workers thought that the formation of lactic acid from glycogen was the fundamental reaction of muscular contraction: oxidation took place a second time to supply the energy for the resynthesis of glycogen from lactic acid, to allow for prolonged activity of the muscle. Without lactic acid no muscular contraction was supposed to be possible.

This, which was called the *Hill–Meyerhof theory* of muscular contraction, was almost universally accepted by physiologists at that time. A 'revolution in muscle physiology', to use A. V. Hill's (1932) terminology, took place in 1930 when a young Danish physiologist, E. Lundsgaard, found that a muscle poisoned with monoiodacetic acid, a substance that prevents lactic acid production, is capable of performing a number of contractions. The only difference from the normal state is that the total number of contractions is very limited in muscle poisoned in this way: the muscle becomes alkaline, instead of acid. The energy for the work performed by the muscle was apparently furnished by the splitting of *creatine phosphate* into its components, a highly exergonic reaction.

The Hill–Meyerhof theory had to be adapted to this new finding: the splitting of creatine phosphate was then considered to be the reaction directly involved in the supply of energy for the performance of mechanical work, thus preceding the glycolytic reaction. This last was simply displaced from the first to the second rank, but it retained its full quantitative significance and importance as a source of chemical energy for muscular contraction.

In particular, lactic acid formation from glycogen was still considered a necessary step in the chain reaction involved in muscular contraction; the complete combustion of glycogen also had to go through lactic acid as a necessary intermediate product. Furthermore, glycolysis was still considered the principal, though an indirect, source of anaerobic energy responsible for muscular contraction, and lactic acid formation from—and resynthesis to—glycogen were considered to be the only mechanisms for the contraction and payment of an oxygen debt.

If this were the case, a relationship should have been found between the amount of lactic acid formed as a consequence of the exercise and the oxygen debt. Furthermore, the kinetics of disappearance of lactic acid from the blood should parallel the oxygen debt payment. In 1933 Margaria, Edwards, and Dill could not confirm these premises. First of all they found that no lactic acid above the resting value was detectable at all at low or moderate grades of work, in spite of a consistent oxygen debt formation: lactic acid appeared in the blood only after strenuous exercise intense enough to call for oxygen consumption close to the maximum. Under such conditions the oxygen debt increased apparently linearly with increasing of lactic acid concentration in the blood (Fig. 1.1).

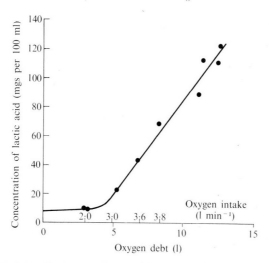

Fig. 1.1. Relationship between lactic acid concentration, oxygen debt as calculated by Hill, and metabolic rate, at steady state of exercise. Duration of exercise was 10 min in each case. (From Margaria, Edwards, and Dill 1933.)

4 Energy sources in muscular exercise

On the other hand, the kinetics of lactic acid disappearance was found to be strikingly different from that of the oxygen debt payment: the first appears to be a simple exponential reaction having a half reaction time of 15 min, whereas the oxygen consumption in recovery appears to be a more complex process in which at least two exponential processes are involved. The first is a fast one, having a half reaction time of 0·5 min; the second is very slow, with a half reaction time of 15 min, of the same order of magnitude as that of lactic acid disappearance (see Fig. 1.2).

It appeared from these data that the metabolism of lactic acid was too slow to account for the intense oxidative processes that take place in the body during muscular exercise: evidently glycogen or other metabolites burned in muscle during activity cannot go through the lactic acid pathway, for this would slow the

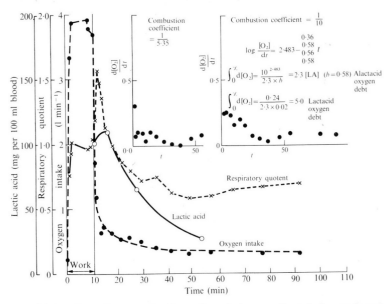

Fig. 1.2. Lactic acid, oxygen intake, and respiratory quotient during work and recovery. The subject was running at a speed of 18·6 km h^{-1} for 10 minutes. The two smaller graphs at the top of the Figure show oxygen consumption per minute during recovery, less the basal oxygen consumption and less the amount attributable to the combustion of the lactic acid as calculated from the disappearance of lactic acid on the assumption of a combustion coefficient of 1/5·35 (left) and 1/10 (right). (From Margaria, Edwards, and Dill 1933.)

whole reaction chain of oxidations to a rate much lower than that actually observed.

Thus the cleavage of glycogen to lactic acid seems to be a process that takes place in muscular exercise only as an emergency mechanism in strenuous exercise. Under these conditions lactic acid formation has in effect the significance of the contraction of an oxygen debt, as A. V. Hill suggested. But the oxygen debt contracted at lower levels of exercise is not due to glycolysis, but to some other anaerobic reactions, which Margaria *et al.* (1933) attributed to creatine phosphate cleavage. A distinction was therefore made between that fraction of oxygen debt due to creatine phosphate cleavage, which was termed 'alactic' and is repaid very rapidly in recovery, and the other fraction, due to glycolysis (*lactacid* oxygen debt), which is repaid much more slowly, as is shown by the kinetics of the disappearance of lactic acid from the blood. The amounts of these two fractions of the oxygen debt are plotted as a function of the oxygen intake in Fig. 1.3.

From these experiments it appeared also that the combustion coefficient of lactic acid, i.e. the fraction of lactic acid burned to supply the energy for its resynthesis to glycogen, was not $\frac{1}{4}$ as Meyerhof had suggested, but much lower. From the disappearance of lactic acid from the blood the oxygen consumption involved could be calculated for a given value of the combustion coefficient: if this value was assumed to be $\frac{1}{4}$, the calculated value of the oxygen consumption involved was higher than the oxygen consumption actually found. A reasonable figure for the combustion coefficient of lactic acid appeared to be not higher than $\frac{1}{8}-\frac{1}{10}$.

A few years later it was found that the cleavage of the creatine phosphate in muscle can take place only in the presence of a compound isolated from muscle by K. Lohman in 1929, *adenosine triphosphate*, which splits into adenosine diphosphate and inorganic phosphate. This is also a reaction yielding a large amount of energy. Adenosine triphosphate or a similar substance is now considered to be the fundamental energy-yielding compound, not only in muscular contraction, but in all biochemical processes that require energy transformation.

The adenosine triphosphate reaction has therefore also been inserted in the chain of reactions taking place in muscular contraction preceding the cleavage of creatine phosphate. This last

8 Energy sources in muscular exercise

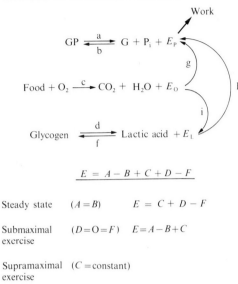

$$E = A - B + C + D - F$$

Steady state $(A = B)$ $E = C + D - F$

Submaximal $(D = 0 = F)$ $E = A - B + C$
exercise

Supramaximal $(C = \text{constant})$
exercise

Fig. 1.4. Scheme of the main energetic reactions that occur in muscular exercise. GP, phosphagen; P, inorganic phosphate; EN, energy involved in the reaction; W, energy transformed into mechanical work. The subscripts indicate the chemical origin of the energy: O, oxygen; P, phosphagen; L, glycolysis.

liberated when 1 g of lactic acid is formed or 1 ml of oxygen is consumed.

Although it has been known for some time that the energy equivalent of 1 ml of oxygen used in the combustion of food amounts to about 5 cal, the energy equivalent of phosphagen, and of lactic acid formed from glycogen in man were not known with accuracy until a short time ago, because measurements had never been made *in vivo* under physiological conditions. Therefore the energy cost of performances in which a prominent part of the energy was derived from the cleavage of phosphagen or from glycolysis could not be known with certainty. Such performances include all maximal efforts of short duration, such as for example the 100-metre or the 400-metre sprints in athletics.

When the energy equivalents of phosphagen, lactic acid, and oxygen are known and an exact energy balance is made, then the two most significant peculiarities of the energetic process, i.e. (a) the *capacity* or the total quantity of energy available, and (b) the *power*, that is the energy transformed in unit time, can be determined for all three processes separately.

The energy from oxidations

The values of the energy equivalents for lactic acid or for oxygen can be obtained by making use of eqn (1.1): this, however, contains too many unknown factors. Some experimental conditions have been devised in which some of the factors can be neglected to obtain a simpler formula. For example, it is known that in submaximal work no production of lactic acid takes place: under such conditions D and F are therefore zero. It is also commonly known that in all types of exercise of constant intensity, after 1 min or less the phosphagen content in the muscles reaches equilibrium, i.e. the same amount of phosphagen is split as is resynthesized. Under these conditions the energy liberated therefore equals that absorbed, or $A = B$.

Thence, in *submaximal work*, i.e. that which requires an oxygen consumption less than the maximum, and under steady-state conditions as defined above, reaction (1.1) can be simplified as

$$E = C = MV_{O_2} \qquad (1.2)$$

where M is the *energy equivalent of* 1 1 *of oxygen*, and V_{O_2} the volume of oxygen consumed in millilitres.

Since, as pointed out above, 1 ml of oxygen used in the combustion of food liberates about 5 cal, i.e. $M = 5$, it is easy to calculate from the oxygen consumption the energy spent for a given work-load. This has been done in physiological work for many years, to obtain the energy cost of an exercise.

The energy equivalent of the glycolytic process

More difficult is the measurement of the energy equivalent of glycolysis, i.e. of lactic acid formation. This analysis can be made only in *supramaximal exercise*, i.e. exercise greater than that which can be met solely by oxidation. The limit to oxidation is apparently set by the maximum amount of oxygen that can be transported to the tissues through the circulation.

In strenuous supramaximal exercise a steady state for phosphagen splitting and resynthesis can be reached within a few seconds, after which, as stated above, $A = B$; as a result these factors disappear from eqn (1.1).

Moreover, the rate of glycogen resynthesis from lactic acid (reaction f) is a very slow process; it is known that it is of an exponential type with a half reaction time of about 15 min (Margaria *et al.* 1933; Margaria and Edwards 1934). When supramaximal exercise lasts only a relatively short period (1–5 min), this reaction can therefore be disregarded. Eqn (1.1) then simplifies to:

$$E = C + D = MV_{O_2}^{max} + N(LA) \qquad (1.3)$$

or

$$\dot{E} = M\dot{V}_{O_2}^{max} + N(\dot{L}A), \qquad (1.4)$$

where $\dot{E}$ is the energy required per min, $\dot{V}_{O_2}^{max}$ the maximum oxygen consumption per min, (LA) the amount of lactic acid produced in 1 minute (in grams), and N is the energy equivalent of lactic acid formation from glycogen.

In supramaximal exercise the oxygen consumption has reached its maximal value $\dot{V}_{O_2}^{max}$, which is constant, independent of the energy requirement; under these conditions, for a given subject the production of lactic acid per min, (LA) should be a linear function of the energy requirement $\dot{E}$. Furthermore, for a given work-load, or energy requirement ($\dot{E}$ = constant), the amount of lactic acid formed, or its concentration in the blood, should also be a linear function of time.

These hypotheses have been proved correct in experiments on man and animals which measured the amount of lactic acid that appeared in the blood during exercise of varying supramaximal intensities, all of which led to exhaustion in 1–10 min.

The collection of the blood samples was, however, a serious problem, because of the difficulty of drawing blood from the vein of a running subject; furthermore, the concentration of lactic acid in the blood during the run would not be indicative of the total quantity of lactic acid formed in the whole body at that instant, because it takes time for the lactic acid to diffuse from the muscles into the body fluids. This difficulty was overcome by having the subject stop after a given period (e.g. 1, 2, or 3 min of work, according to the intensity of the exercise), and by taking the blood samples 2–3 min afterwards, in order to allow the lactic acid to reach a uniform distribution in all body fluids. Only when these conditions were satisfied was the concentration of lactic acid in the blood representative of the total quantity of lactic acid formed.

The data obtained in a series of experiments conducted at four different work-loads (Margaria, Cerretelli, di Prampero, Massari,

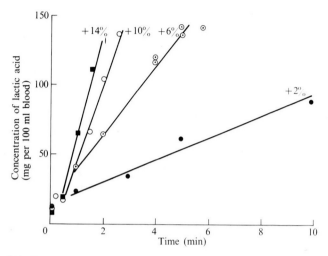

Fig. 1.5. The concentration of lactic acid in the blood in supramaximal work (running at a constant speed of 12 km h^{-1} on a treadmill at gradients changing from +2 per cent to +14 per cent as indicated) increases linearly with the duration of the performance. The rate of increase is linearly related with the intensity of the exercise (see Fig. 1.6). (From Margaria *et al.* 1963.)

and Torelli 1963*b*) are summarized in Fig. 1.5; those from other sets of experiments are shown in Figs 1.7 and 1.8. All these results lead to the conclusion that for a given work-load the concentration of lactic acid in the blood increases linearly with time, as predicted.

From the concentration of lactic acid in the blood the amount (in grams) of lactic acid produced in the whole body can be calculated when the body weight is known; certain assumptions are made about the distribution of lactic acid in all organs and tissues. The lactic acid produced per minute and per kilogram of body weight is shown in Fig. 1.6 as a function of the energy requirement: this function also appears to be linear, as predicted by eqn (1.4). The line cuts the abscissa at the point where energy expenditure is equal to the maximum oxygen consumption.

The left-hand ordinate of Fig. 1.6 refers to the oxygen consumption, which in submaximal work increases linearly with the energy requirement, according to eqn (1.2), reaching a maximal constant value ($\dot{V}_{O_2}^{max}$) when the energy requirement, exceeds a given limiting value. This indicates that in steady-state exercise the body normally meets the energy requirement exclusively by oxidations; only when these cannot cope with the energy expenditure, as in supramaximal work, does glycolysis enter into play as an additional emergency mechanism. This statement is important, for it gives a precise quantitative significance to lactic acid formation in exercise.

The energy equivalent of lactic acid formation from glycogen

The slope of the lactic acid line in Fig. 1.6 is an index of the energy liberated per gram of lactic acid formed from glycogen: it is in fact, as from eqn (1.4), $dE/d(LA) = N$. It amounts to about 230 cal per g and it is independent of the amount of lactic acid formed or of the intensity of the exercise. This thermodynamic value appears to be particularly significant and reliable, for it is

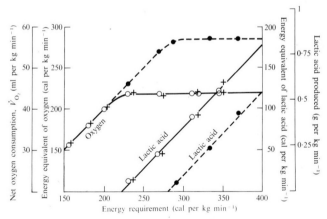

Fig. 1.6. Rate of lactic acid production (g min^{-1}) as an effect of the exercise (ordinate at right) are plotted as a function of the work intensity and, therefore, of the energy requirement (abscissa). A straight line is obtained that cuts the abscissa at an energy requirement corresponding to 220 cal per kg min^{-1}; below this value no production of lactic acid takes place and the energy requirement is met solely by oxygen consumption (shown on the ordinate at left).
The broken lines refer to athletes (middle- and long-distance runners) whose maximum oxygen consumption is higher; the line of the lactic acid for these subjects is correspondingly shifted to the right. (From Margaria *et al.* 1963.)

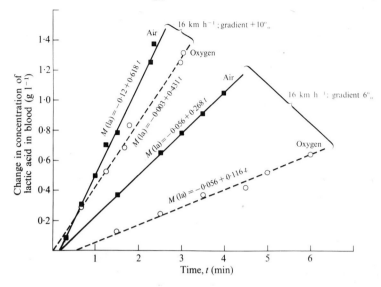

Fig. 1.7. Blood lactic acid $(g\ l^{-1})$ above the rest value as a function of the time of performance in two exercises of different intensities: during the performance the subject was breathing air or pure oxygen. The regression lines have been calculated with the method of least squares. (From Margaria *et al.* 1972.)

obtained *in vivo* in man under perfect physiological conditions, i.e. at a temperature of 37 °C, at the pH, osmotic pressure, ionic strength, etc. of the body fluids.

Athletes (long- or middle-distance runners) differ from ordinary people by having an appreciably greater maximum oxygen consumption. In them also lactic acid formation takes place only when the energy requirement is greater than can be met by oxidation: the lactic acid line of Fig. 1.6 is therefore shifted to the right; its slope is obviously the same, for it has the significance of a thermodynamic constant, the *energy equivalent of lactic acid*.

The effect of work-load on the rate of lactic acid appearance in blood is shown in Fig. 1.7 for a subject running on a treadmill at 16 km h^{-1} at two different gradients as indicated, when breathing either air or pure oxygen. For each of the two sets of data, the total energy requirement $\dot{E}$ is known, and the lactic acid production per minute, $\dot{M}(LA)$, is given by the slopes of the lines in Fig. 1.7. The two values of $\dot{V}_{O_2}^{max}$ can also be calculated, together with the constant N, the energy equivalent of lactic acid, by making use of eqn (1.4). It turns out that N has a value of 240 cal per g, which is close to that obtained from the experiments described in Figs 1.5 and 1.6.

When the subject breathes pure oxygen the maximal oxygen consumption increases and the lactic acid production is correspondingly decreased (Fig. 1.7): the condition approaches that of the athlete. The increase is about 9 per cent, approximately the same as the increase in oxygen content of the arterial blood due to the higher amount of the physically dissolved oxygen, and to the corresponding higher volume of oxygen transported to the muscles for an unchanged volume pumped by the heart per minute. This seems to indicate that the limit to maximal oxygen consumption is set by the amount of oxygen that can reach the muscles and not by factors intrinsic in the muscles.

Here I would like to mention the effect of breathing oxygen during the actual performance of work: in some sporting events oxygen is given to the athletes in the intervals between games, but this practice is of no use and it has no physiological basis.

On the other hand, in *anoxia*, which can be induced experimentally by breathing a mixture deficient in oxygen, or at high altitude (such at Mexico City, where the 1968 Olympic Games were held), the maximum oxygen consumption decreases, and the performance of aerobic work is reduced. Correspondingly, the line of lactic acid production is shifted to the left; its slope, however, maintains the same value under all conditions.

The validity of eqn (1.4) can also be tested by maintaining a constant work-load and varying the maximum oxygen consumption by using subjects of different capacities to perform aerobic work. The production of lactic acid per minute is then higher the lower the maximum oxygen consumption of the subject (Fig. 1.8). By plotting the lactic acid production per minute against $V_{O_2}^{max}$ for all the subjects tested, a straight line is again obtained (Fig. 1.9): its slope represents the energy equivalent for lactic acid, expressed in volume of oxygen, instead of calories, as above: the value amounts to 49 ml of oxygen (or 245 calories) per gram of lactic acid, a value not too different from that obtained in the first series of experiments.

Other data from the literature lead to the same value for the energy equivalent of lactic acid. In 1934, Margaria and Edwards performed the following experiment. A subject made successive

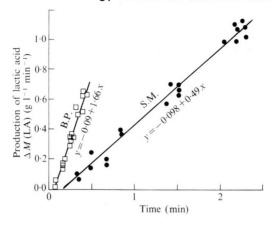

Fig. 1.8. The lactic acid concentration in the blood increases linearly with the duration of the exercise (running on a treadmill at 16 km h^{-1} and an incline of 10 per cent). The slope of the line, that is the lactic acid production per minute, is much greater in the non-athlete than in the athlete, who has an anaerobic power more than twice as great. (From Margaria *et al.* 1972.)

very strenuous runs to exhaustion on a treadmill at 18·7 km h^{-1} on an 11·5 per cent incline at intervals of 5 min; the blood lactic acid was measured immediately before and after each run. The increase in lactic acid as a result of each run was plotted against the time to exhaustion of each performance, which amounted to a

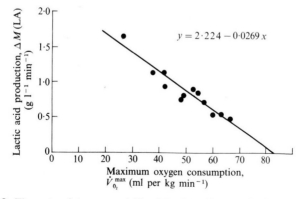

Fig. 1.9. The rate of increase of blood lactic acid per min for 12 subjects, including the two of Fig. 1.8, all performing the same exercise, is plotted as a function of their maximum aerobic power. The slope of the line is an index of the energy equivalent of lactic acid (see text). (From Margaria *et al.* 1972.)

maximum, of 35 s, in the first run. This time decreased progressively in the successive runs together with the decreased capacity of the body to produce lactic acid: the increase in lactic acid concentration during the first run was about 100 mg per 100 ml; during the second about 25 mg per 100 ml; and during the third 0–5 mg per 100 ml (Margaria and Edwards 1934). These data are given in Fig. 1.10 as a function of the duration of the run. The function appears to be a straight line defined by the equation

$$\Delta(LA) = -65 \cdot 9 + 4 \cdot 33 s,$$

where $\Delta(LA)$ denotes the change in the concentration of lactic acid in the blood (mg per 100 ml) and s is the time to exhaustion, in seconds. The energy cost of such exercise was found to be 8·2 cal per kg s^{-1} (Margaria, Cerretelli, Aghemo, and Sassi 1963a). The function can be plotted as a function of the energy expended (in cal per kg) and the weight of lactic acid (in grams) per kg of body weight can be substituted for the lactic acid concentration in the blood. The equation in this case appears to be

$$(LA)(g \text{ per kg}) = -0 \cdot 494 + 0 \cdot 00396 \, E(\text{cal per kg}),$$

from which $dE/d(LA)$ of lactic acid can be calculated as about 250 cal g^{-1}.

A value of 248 ± 32 cal g^{-1} for the energy equivalent of lactic

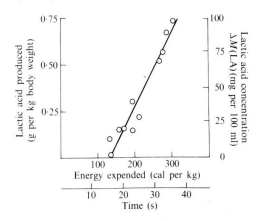

Fig. 1.10. Lactic acid produced as a function of the energy expended in a strenuous supramaximal exercise (calculated from the data of Margaria and Edwards (1934); from Margaria (1963)).

acid formed from glycogen in the muscles has been obtained by Cerretelli and others using a gastrocnemius muscle preparation of the dog (Cerretelli, di Prampero, and Piiper 1969). This result was reached without making any assumption about the distribution of lactic acid between tissues and body fluids, for the total lactic acid produced was measured directly in the muscle or in the blood flowing through it. The identity of the two figures obtained in man and in the isolated muscle indicates that the assumptions concerning the lactic acid distribution in the body fluids at equilibrium in man were approximately correct, given the particular body composition of the subjects of the experiments.

It is, however, possible that such distribution varies appreciably from subject to subject according to the chemical composition of the body, and particularly its fat content.

By mixing oil with a solution of lactic acid in water and shaking until an equilibrium is reached, the partition coefficient of lactic acid between water and fat can be determined. It has been found that only a very small fraction of the lactic acid leaves the watery phase to pass into the fat. Similarly, if the same amount of lactic acid is injected in two animals of very different fat content, but of the same lean body weight, the concentration of lactic acid in the blood is about the same. Therefore when converting the lactic acid concentration in the blood to the amount of lactic acid per kilogram of body weight, due allowance should be made for the fat content of the body.

Calculation of the maximum aerobic power from blood lactic acid

Since the slope of the lines relating lactic acid production per minute with energy requirement in supramaximal exercise (Fig. 1.6) is constant under all conditions, and since the lines cut the abscissa at a value of energy requirement coinciding with the *maximum aerobic power* in calories per kilogram body weight of the subject, a single determination of the lactic acid production in supramaximum exercise is sufficient to calculate the maximum aerobic power. In fact, as shown in Figs 1.5 and 1.7, the lactic acid starts to increase very soon after the beginning of the exercise ($t = 0$). The rate of increase in lactic acid concentration in the blood is obtained by dividing the lactic acid found in the blood after a given time of supramaximal exercise by the duration of the performance. This is converted into grams of lactic acid produced per kilogram of body weight per minute. This figure can be multiplied by the *energy coefficient of lactic acid*, 240 cal g^{-1}, to obtain the energy spent per minute due to lactic acid formation. The maximum aerobic power can then be easily obtained by subtracting this value from the total energy requirement for the particular exercise, as given by eqn (1.4).

This is possibly as good a method for measuring the maximum aerobic power as the direct one, and it is to be preferred when there are no facilities for measuring oxygen consumption. An advantage of this procedure is that it is not necessary to rush the subject to exhaustion. For example, with a subject running at 16 km h^{-1} on a 6 per cent incline and breathing air (see Fig. 1.7) it should suffice to take the blood sample after 3 min of running. The increase in blood lactic acid as a result of the run amounts to 0.8 g l^{-1} or 0.267 g l^{-1} min^{-1}, which corresponds to 0.20 g min^{-1} per kg. The calorific equivalent of this amount of lactic acid is $240 \times 0.20 = 48$ cal per kg min^{-1}. As the energy requirement for this exercise is 340 cal per kg min^{-1} (Margaria, Cerretelli, and Mangili 1964) the aerobic power of the subject is $340 - 48 = 292$ cal, or 58.4 ml of oxygen per kilogram of body weight per minute.

Lactic acid in submaximal exercise

While Fig. 1.6 indicates that no appreciable production of lactic acid takes place in submaximal exercise, lactic acid may also be found in blood at work-loads entailing an oxygen consumption as low as 60–70 per cent of the maximum. From these observations some authors have inferred that the glycolytic process also plays a significant role at submaximal work levels (Astrand, Cliddy, Saltin, and Stenberg 1964; Rowell, Blackman, Martin, Mazzarella, and Bruce 1965; Hermansen and Saltin 1967). The discrepancy could possibly be explained by assuming that the oxidative processes in muscle are rather sluggish, and that it takes several seconds or a few minutes from the onset of the exercise to reach an oxygen consumption that can keep pace with the energy demand. In this phase the working muscles reach a condition of relative anoxia, during which lactic acid is produced. This, however, should be only a temporary affair, lasting only until the

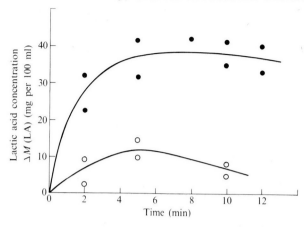

Fig. 1.11. Lactic acid concentration in blood (mg per 100 ml) as a function of the duration of the exercise. The work-load expressed as a percentage of the maximum aerobic power was 70–80 (open circles) and 90–100 (closed circles). Subject non-athletic. (From Saiki, Margaria, and Cuttica 1967.)

oxidative processes are fully at work to meet the energy requirement; after this condition is reached, and the steady-state oxygen consumption has been attained, lactic acid should increase no further, or possibly even disappear from the blood.

Experiments showed that this is in fact the case: in a subject performing at 90–100 per cent or 70–80 per cent of his maximum oxygen consumption, lactic acid increased in the blood in the first 2–3 min, after which it became constant or even decreased toward its original rest values (Fig. 1.11).

The lactic acid found in blood after a few minutes of submaximal exercise cannot therefore be taken as an indication that a glycolytic process is active during steady-state exercise. Its persistence in the blood even after several minutes of exercise is due to the characteristically slow removal of the lactic acid formed at the onset of exercise.

To plot on the same graph two substantially different curves, one indicative of power ($\dot{V}_{O_2}$) and the other indicative of energy (blood lactic acid) is obviously misleading: if lactic acid data are converted into power units by taking the increase of lactic acid per minute in a significant time-interval at steady state, the error is avoided (Saiki, Margaria, and Cuttica 1967).

Capacity and power of the glycolytic mechanism

Once the value of the calorific coefficient of lactic acid is known, the capacity of this mechanism is easily found. It is well known that the maximum increase of lactic acid in blood as a result of strenuous muscular exercise amounts to about 1·5 g l⁻¹, or to about 1·12 grams per kilogram of body weight. The maximum quantity of energy obtainable from the formation of lactic acid is thus about 270 cal per kilogram of body weight, corresponding to about 54 ml of oxygen, a value somewhat greater than the maximal oxygen consumption in 1 min.

It has been mentioned above that the oxygen consumption increases in parallel with the energy requirement up to a limit that is presumably set by the maximum quantity of oxygen that can be transported by the blood to the active muscles. The amount of lactic acid that can be produced per minute also presumably has an upper limit, which is set by the maximum speed of the chemical processes involved in its production from glycogen: in fact, as the work intensity is progressively increased beyond a determined level, the lactic acid produced per minute does not increase further (as is indicated by the slopes of the lines

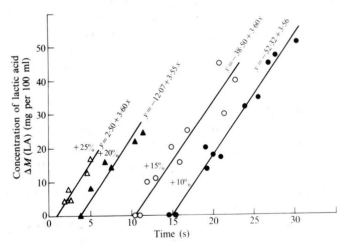

Fig. 1.12. Concentration of lactic acid in blood in supramaximal exercise. The four lines refer to four different work-loads, consisting of running on a treadmill at a constant speed of 18 km h⁻¹, but at an incline increasing from 10 per cent to 25 per cent, as indicated. Each line ends at the time corresponding to exhaustion.
(From Margaria *et al.* 1964.)

in Fig. 1.12, which appear to be the same, and independent of the work-load). This maximum value of lactic acid production may then be taken as indicative of the *maximum power* of this process: it amounts to approximately $1 \cdot 7$ per kg min^{-1}, which corresponds to a power of about 410 cal per kg min^{-1}, or to an oxygen consumption of 82 ml per kg min^{-1}, which is about twice as great as the power due to oxidation alone.

Capacity and power of the alactic mechanism

In very strenuous exercise, such as running at 18 km h^{-1} on a 10 per cent incline, which calls for a maximum rate of lactic acid production, a condition of exhaustion is reached in about 30–40 s. It is interesting to note that, despite the severity of the exercise, no lactic acid is produced at its onset (Margaria *et al.* 1964): as shown in Fig. 1.12, in the mildest exercise of the set (line at the extreme right), lactic acid does not in fact appear until after about 15 s from the beginning of the exercise. In this initial phase, then, the glycolytic mechanism does not contribute at all to the energy balance; on the other hand, the oxidative mechanism is rather sluggish, and during the first few seconds of exercise can participate only to a very minor extent.

It appears from previous experiments (Margaria *et al.* 1965) that at the onset of strenuous exercise the oxygen consumption increases exponentially, the rate of increase depending on the intensity of the exercise (Fig. 1.13). The half reaction time of this process is about 30 s.

The oxygen consumption in the experiments shown in Fig. 1.12 was then calculated, and the corresponding energy subtracted from the total energy expenditure to obtain the net energy due to the anaerobic processes involved in the exercise.

In Fig. 1.14 the duration of each of the experiments described in Fig. 1.12 is plotted against the work-load or power, as given by the energy requirement. The duration of the work accomplished before any lactic acid formation took place is also plotted ('alac-tic'), also shown corrected by the oxygen consumed in that period ('corrected alactic'). This last line refers to the work due solely to phosphagen cleavage. It is apparent that the higher the work-load the shorter is the duration of the exercise.

By extrapolating the line to $t = 0$ we can determine the *maximum power* which can be exploited in very short-lasting exercise.

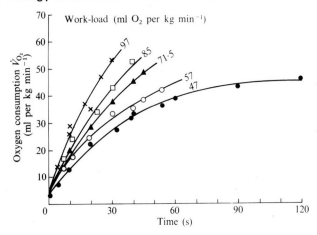

Fig. 1.13. Oxygen consumption at the onset of exercise at different work-loads, expressed as oxygen requirement as indicated. (From Margaria *et al.* 1965.)

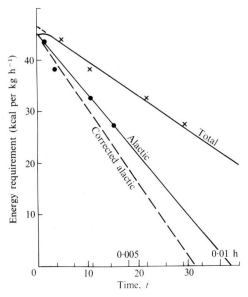

Fig. 1.14. Time of performance in seconds or in hours for a work-load of a given intensity. The time for which the exercise can be sustained without any lactic acid formation, as from the data of Fig. 1.12, is also indicated 'alactic': by subtracting the energy sustained by oxidative processes taking place in the first few seconds of exercise the line 'corrected alactic' is obtained. (From Margaria *et al.* 1964.)

This is obviously due to phosphagen cleavage only, and it amounts in our subjects to about 50 kcal per kg h^{-1}, a value about three times as high as the *maximum aerobic power*, which amounted in our subjects to 42 ml of oxygen per kilogram per minute or to about 13 kcal per kg h^{-1}.

The four points defining the function 'alactic' of Fig. 1.14 are roughly on a straight line. Assuming that this function is also approximately linear for all the values of power and duration of the performance, then the area delimited by the line and the axes represents the potential maximum amount of energy obtained from this process. This area is in fact the integral of the power with respect to the duration: for the data of Fig. 1.14 it corresponds to 196 cal, or about 40 ml of oxygen per kilogram of body weight, expressed in terms of oxygen requirement.

As the efficiency of phosphagen resynthesis by oxidation is about 0·60, then the maximum anaerobic energy expressed in terms of phosphagen cleavage is $196 \times 0·60 = 117·6$ cal per kg of body weight. Assuming now that the muscles involved in running are about 40 per cent of the body mass, the energy from phosphagen amounts to $117·6/0·40 = 294$ cal per kilogram of muscle: and assuming further that the energy equivalent of phosphagen is the same as for creatine phosphate, 11 000 cal mol^{-1} (Wilkie 1968), the phosphagen content of the skeletal muscles turns out to be 27 mM per kg. This figure is not too far from that obtained from chemical determinations in man and animals (Lohmann 1934; Bergström 1967; Hultman, Bergström, and McLennan Anderson 1967; Karlsson 1971).

In Fig. 1.15 the power developed by each of the three processes, oxidative, alactic, and lactic, is plotted as a function of the time from the start of the exercise (not as a function of the time to exhaustion as in Fig. 1.14). The areas indicated represent the amounts of energy contributed by the three processes separately. These curves have been drawn on the assumption that all the lactic acid production resulting from the exercise took place during the actual performance of the exercise. The possibility that at least a fraction of it may have been formed after the end of the exercise, in the first phase of recovery, is a real one, as it will be shown later, and it provides an explanation for the excess energy that appears to be spent towards the end of the least strenuous exercise (indicated by the shaded area below the abscissa). This

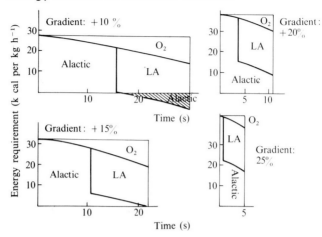

Fig. 1.15. The power developed by the three processes, oxidative, alactic, and lactic, in exercises to exhaustion at different intensity. The energy requirement of the exercise is indicated by the height of the upper horizontal line. The duration of the exercise is indicated by the end of the graph. The areas labelled O_2, Alactic, and LA indicate the energy contribution of each of the three mechanisms. This figure was constructed from the experimental data of Fig. 1.12. (From Margaria *et al.* 1964.)

probably corresponds to an amount of lactic acid formed after the end of the exercise, its energy being utilized to pay a corresponding amount of the alactic oxygen debt contracted in the initial phase of the exercise.

Presumably, for the other three more strenuous exercises the amount of alactic oxygen debt contracted—and therefore of the phosphagen actually split during the exercise—is also greater than it appears to be from the graphs; the fraction of lactic acid produced in recovery was probably even greater, since the workload was greater and the time to exhaustion shorter.

The maximum amount of energy liberated by the alactic mechanism in these experiments, shown by the relevant areas in Fig. 1.15, amounts to about 100 cal per kg, corresponding to an alactic oxygen debt of 20 ml per kg. This is about the same as the oxygen debt actually measured from the oxygen consumption curve at the end of a maximal exercise (Margaria and Edwards 1934; di Prampero, Peeters, and Margaria 1973). It seems that in maximal exercise only a fraction, about half, of the phosphagen contained in the muscle can be made available for the contraction of an oxygen debt. In supramaximal exercise, however, a much larger amount of phosphagen may be split, which does not all appear as alactic oxygen debt during recovery, this being paid by the production of lactic acid in the 2–3 min interval between the end of the exercise and the collection of the blood sample. The *actual capacity of this mechanism* is therefore probably appreciably greater than the 20 ml indicated.

More recently the kinetics of oxygen consumption has been measured in man on a breath-by-breath basis during recovery from very strenuous supramaximal exercise leading to exhaustion in 10–50 s (di Prampero *et al.* 1973). It was found that the oxygen consumption does not decrease immediately at the end of the exercise, as it does after maximal or submaximal aerobic exercise: it remains at the maximal level for a short time (12–35 s). The subsequent decrease follows a trend similar to that observed after aerobic exercise, and the kinetics is similar: i.e. the half reaction time is 25–30 s (Fig. 1.16).

In Fig. 1.16 two recovery oxygen consumption curves are shown, one (on the left) after maximal exercise, the other (right) after supramaximal exercise. Evidently in maximal exercise the oxygen debt is given simply by the integral of the exponential function, starting from the maximum oxygen consumption, and it amounts to about 20 ml of oxygen. For supramaximal exercise an additional amount of oxygen consumed during the first 0·5 min of recovery at the maximum oxygen consumption level, amounting to about 15 ml, must be added, so raising the total alactic oxygen debt to 35 ml.

It is not surprising that the oxygen consumption in recovery following supramaximal exercise stays at the maximum level for a few seconds as presumably the level of the oxidative processes in muscle is dependent on the level of split phosphagen in muscle. In maximal aerobic exercise the amount of split phosphagen in the muscles is kept constant because the rate of phosphagen cleavage can just be met by the rate of phosphagen resynthesis due to oxidation; when at the end of the exercise phosphagen cleavage suddenly stops, while phosphagen resynthesis proceeds, the amount of split phosphagen, and consequently also the oxygen consumption in the muscles decreases immediately.

In supramaximal exercise the rate of phosphagen resynthesis, which is limited by the maximal rate of oxygen consumption (and

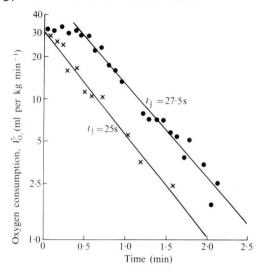

Fig. 1.16. Semi-logarithmic plot of oxygen uptake (ml per kg min^{-1}) in recovery after steady-state maximal aerobic exercise (run at 12 km h^{-1}; incline 2 per cent) (crosses) and after 11 s of supramaximal exercise to exhaustion (18 km h^{-1}; 20 per cent) (circles). Data indicating alactic oxygen debt payment are obtained by subtracting from oxygen uptake in recovery the amount due to the slow component, as obtained from graphical back-extrapolation of the single exponential regression line through the oxygen uptake data obtained from 3 to 15 min of recovery. Supramaximal exercise was started from a steady-state aerobic exercise involving a oxygen consumption 50 per cent of the maximal; circles indicate average value of four runs on one subject. (From di Prampero *et al.* 1973.)

lactic acid production) cannot cope with the rate of phosphagen splitting. As a result, a much higher concentration of split phosphagen in the muscles is reached. At the end of the exercise oxidation will therefore take place at the maximal rate until the split phosphagen in the muscles has been reduced to the critical level corresponding to the maximum oxygen consumption: only thereafter will the oxygen consumption decrease in parallel with the resynthesis of phosphagen. This explanation is based on the hypothesis that the intensity of the oxidations in muscle is dictated by the level of split phosphagen.

Though the mechanism of the regulation of oxygen consumption during exercise is not well understood, this hypothesis seems to me very tenable, in view of the fact that cleavage of high-energy phosphate compounds leads to a lowering of the oxidation potential in the tissues, thus promoting the reduction of oxygen or other substrates that are susceptible to being converted from a more oxidized to a more reduced state.

Presumably this is also the case for the pyruvate–lactate system, and it provides the explanation for the accumulation of lactate in strenuous supramaximal exercise when oxidation cannot keep pace with phosphagen cleavage.

If the exercise is extremely strenuous, so as to lead to exhaustion in a very short time, that is insufficient for the oxygen consumption to reach a maximal level, then oxygen consumption continues to increase during the first few seconds of recovery after the exercise is over. It does not fall until after it has reached the maximal value, and then the usual kinetics applies.

That the rate of oxygen uptake is conditioned by the amount of split phosphagen in the muscles also seems to be suggested by the finding by Margaria *et al.* (1933) that the amount of the alactic oxygen debt is linearly related to the steady-state oxygen consumption (Fig. 1.3). The alactic oxygen debt in this condition is evidently the expression of the oxidative energy necessary to resynthesize the split phosphagen and must be proportional to it. This linear relation is obviously valid only up to the maximum value of oxygen consumption, which appears to be limited by the capacity for oxygen transport to the active tissues: above that value, a further increase in the split phosphagen in muscle cannot lead to increased oxygen consumption.

Anaerobic recovery

A further fraction of the alactic oxygen debt that escapes observation when this is limited to the measurement of the excess oxygen consumption in the first phase of recovery is that paid by delayed lactic acid formation. The energy liberated in the glycolytic process is used in the resynthesis of phosphagen as described by the reactions d, h, and b of the scheme shown in Fig. 1.4: if this takes place in recovery the alactic oxygen debt will be correspondingly reduced. In other words, a lactacid oxygen debt is contracted to contribute to the alactic oxygen debt payment: there is a shift from the alactic to the lactacid oxygen debt.

If recovery is fundamentally visualized as the resynthesis of phosphagen, the primary energy source in muscle activity, this process can be considered as an *anaerobic recovery*. The process of anaerobic recovery was described by Margaria and Moruzzi in 1937 and more recently by Ambrosoli and Cerretelli (1970). If cleavage of glycogen into lactic acid is prevented by poisoning the muscle with monoiodacetic acid, no such recovery takes place (Fig. 1.17).

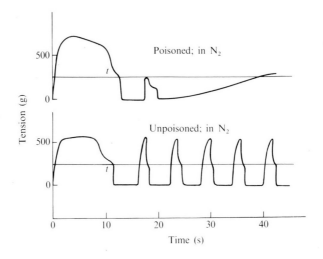

Fig. 1.17. Isometric tetanic contractions of two isolated frog gastrocnemius in nitrogen. The upper tracing is from a monoiodacetate-poisoned frog. The stimulus was maintained until the tension fell to half the value recorded in a single twitch, after which 5 s of rest were allowed before stimulation was resumed. In the unpoisoned muscle the tension after the period of rest is always much higher than at the end of the previous stimulation period: the poisoned muscle on the contrary does not show this 'recovery'. The typical contracture of the poisoned muscle at exhaustion is also evident. (Margaria and Moruzzi 1937.)

The experiments illustrated in Fig. 1.17 show that lactic acid formation can in fact take place during recovery after the exercise is over. This was demonstrated for isolated frog muscle by Embden as early as 1925. Indirect measurements on human subjects have been made by di Prampero *et al.* (1973); lactic acid formation appears to depend on the duration and on the intensity of the supramaximal exercise. The amount of this delayed lactic acid correspond to an oxygen debt of about 10 ml per kilogram of body weight and it may account for about half the total lactic acid produced in short bursts of very violent exercise.

Possible variations of the capacity and power of the alactic mechanism

In conclusion, it appears that although in maximal aerobic steady-state exercise only about half the muscle phosphagen is split, corresponding to an oxygen debt of 20 ml per kilogram of body weight, in strenuous exercise all the phosphagen is made available as an anaerobic source of energy, this being equivalent to an oxygen debt of about 40 ml per kilogram of body weight.

As the energy used in the alactic process comes from phosphagen, it may be predicted that if the unsplit phosphagen content of muscle is decreased, as in steady exercise, both the power and the total energy available from phosphagen cleavage are correspondingly decreased.

This was actually found by Margaria, di Prampero, Aghemo, Derevenco, and Mariani (1971): in young, fit subjects the maximal anaerobic power due to phosphagen breakdown as well as the total energy obtained from the alactic process is decreased when short bursts of very strenuous exercise are performed starting not from a condition of rest but of steady exercise. The power due to phosphagen breakdown is found to be decreased to about half in subjects performing steady exercise at the maximal oxygen consumption level.

This explains the fact that the final sprint in a long race cannot be performed at the same speed as when starting from rest, as in the 100-metre race.

The oxygen debt

The scheme shown in Fig. 1.4, besides describing the energy transformations that take place in the working muscle, illustrates the significance and the characteristics with duration of exercise of the contraction and payment of the *oxygen debt*. As is well known, this term was introduced by A. V. Hill in the 1920s to indicate the energy spent at the beginning of exercise which does not appear as oxygen consumption (*contraction of the oxygen debt*), and which is therefore due to anaerobic reversible processes (reactions a and d in Fig. 1.4). To restore the original chemical condition of the muscle, extra oxygen must be consumed after the period of exercise (*payment of the debt*).

As mentioned earlier, Margaria *et al.* (1933) at the Fatigue Laboratory in Boston found that the oxygen debt is not solely due to lactic acid formation from glycogen, as A. V. Hill suggested. A considerable proportion is due to phosphagen cleavage. This was referred to as the *alactic oxygen debt*, while the fraction due to glycolysis was called the *lactacid debt.*

Since oxidative processes necessarily take place some time after phosphagen cleavage, a certain amount of split phosphagen always exists in active muscles during steady-state exercise. The alactic debt is the amount of oxygen necessary to resynthesize this phosphagen. It will obviously increase with increasing energy demand, i.e. with the intensity of the exercise, as indicated in Fig. 1.3.

The chain reaction c–g–b of Fig. 1.4 that takes place in the first phase of recovery is the expression of the payment of the alactic oxygen debt by oxidations. In supramaximal exercise some of the alactic debt is also paid by the other anaerobic reaction, i.e. lactic acid formation from glycogen (reaction chain d–h–b), but this entails the contraction of an oxygen debt of a different kind: the lactacid one. The payment of the lactacid oxygen debt through the chain reaction c–i–f is a very slow process, as mentioned earlier, because of the slow rate of reaction f.

The measurement of the oxygen debt

Generally the oxygen debt is measured as the total amount of oxygen used during the recovery phase above the rest oxygen consumption value, as suggested by A. V. Hill. This method may, however, lead to a considerable error. It is based on the assumption that the rest oxygen consumption is constant, and that it is not modified by the previous muscular activity; but it is well known that after long strenuous exercise the oxygen consumption does not drop back to the pre-exercise level even after hours, long after the end of any possible oxygen debt payment. Margaria *et al.* (1933) suggested that heavy or prolonged exercise leads to a disturbance of the whole body metabolism and to an increased oxygen consumption that is in no way related to the anaerobic energy spent during the exercise.

The two fractions of the oxygen debt, alactic and lactacid, can most simply be measured separately by making use of the very different kinetics of the two processes. The slow process of the oxygen debt payment is extrapolated to zero recovery time by neglecting the data of the first 4 to 5 min, that is, the alactic oxygen debt, which is paid completely in a very few minutes, can be visualized separately and its amount and kinetics studied.

As the payment of the lactacid oxygen debt must be accompanied by the disappearance of lactate from the blood in recovery, their kinetics are the same. The *amount of the lactacid fraction of the oxygen debt* can easily be calculated from the total amount of lactic acid at the end of the exercise, once the calorific equivalent of lactic acid is known.

The capacity and the kinetics of both fractions of the oxygen debt are obviously strictly related to the energy balance of the two anaerobic systems in Fig. 1.4.

The alactic oxygen debt

This can be visualized as the amount of oxidative energy E_O necessary to resynthesize the split phosphagen, G, that is present in the muscles at the end of the performance. During exercise, as mentioned above, the amount of split phosphagen under steady-state conditions is greater than at rest; it also increases with the work-load. This follows from the fact that the rate of phosphagen breakdown (reaction a in Fig. 1.4) is proportional to the work-load, and therefore to the energy expenditure or to the oxygen requirement $\dot{V}_{O_2}$. Phosphagen cleavage, the fundamental reaction of muscular contraction, is regulated by nervous impulses impinging on the muscles. For a constant work-load the rate of phosphagen cleavage, $-d[G]/dt$ is therefore constant.

On the other hand, reaction b, the resynthesis of phosphagen, is independent of nervous impulses, and according to the law of mass action its rate $d[GP]/dt$ will depend only on the concentration of split phosphagen $[G]$; it will therefore be given by the equations:

$$-\frac{d[GP]}{dt} = a\dot{V}_{O_2} \quad \text{and} \quad \frac{d[GP]}{dt} = k[G] \tag{1.5}$$

where $a = [GP]/\dot{V}_{O_2}$ is a proportionality constant and k is the velocity constant of reaction b.

Under steady-state conditions the rate at which the phosphagen is resynthesized (coupled reactions b and c) is the same as the rate at which it is split: a condition of equilibrium is then reached, which is defined by:

$$a\dot{V}_{O_2} = k[G] \quad \text{and} \quad \dot{V}_{O_2} = k\frac{[G]}{a}. \tag{1.6}$$

As from (1.5) a is the number of moles of phosphagen that can be resynthesized by 1 l of oxygen used in oxidation; $[G]/a$ therefore denotes the alactic oxygen debt, $V_{O_2}^{al}$. It is then:

$$\dot{V}_{O_2} = kV_{O_2}^{al}. \tag{1.7}$$

From eqn (1.7) it appears that the alactic fraction of the oxygen debt should be a linear function of the oxygen consumption, as was actually found in 1933 by Margaria *et al.* (see Fig. 1.3).

Furthermore the slope of this line as defined by the ratio $\dot{V}_{O_2}/V_{O_2}^{al}$ is k, the rate constant for the resynthesis of phosphagen (Margaria 1967). This provides a method for measuring *in vivo* the rate constant of the phosphagen resynthesis process in man under most physiological conditions.

The resynthesis of phosphagen should take place at the same rate as the oxygen debt payment. This has been shown to be an exponential reaction with a half reaction time of about 30 s (Margaria *et al.* 1933); the value of k from the data of Fig. 1.3 is 1·5, which corresponds to a half reaction time of $0·7/1·5 = 0·46$ min or 28 s, almost the same value as that measured directly.

Net and gross alactic oxygen debt. The kinetics of the alactic oxygen debt payment

The oxygen debt as measured by Margaria *et al.* (1933) is the oxygen debt of the entire body (*gross oxygen debt*), and not simply the amount of oxygen necessary to resynthesize the split phosphagen according to the coupled reactions b and c (*net oxygen debt*) (Margaria 1969). In addition the gross alactic debt includes: (1) an amount of oxygen that has been drawn from the stores of the body and has been used up by the muscles, escaping conventional measurement by the analysis of the respiratory gas exchanges; and (2) the oxygen used by the residual activity of muscles not directly involved in the performance of external work, as are the heart and the respiratory muscles.

The oxygen drawn from the stores at maximum oxygen consumption can be estimated by assuming that (a) the saturation of haemoglobin with oxygen of the venous blood is about 55 per cent less than at rest (venous $HbO_2 = 20$ per cent of Hb instead of 75 per cent); (b) the volume of venous blood is 80 per cent of the total blood volume; and (c) the myoglobin, the concentration of which in the muscles is about 2 g per kg, is completely desaturated of oxygen in maximal or supramaximal exercise, but in rest it is completely saturated. The depletion of oxygen stores in maximal exercise can therefore be calculated as amounting to about 0·550 l.

Making this correction to the data in Fig. 1.3 that refer to maximum oxygen consumption, we have

$$k = \frac{\dot{V}_{O_2}^{max} - \dot{V}_{O_2}^{rest}}{\dot{V}_{O_2}^{al} - V^{stores}} = \frac{3 \cdot 9 - 0 \cdot 25}{2 \cdot 5 - 0 \cdot 55} = 1 \cdot 87,$$

$0 \cdot 25$ l min^{-1} being the rest oxygen consumption for this subject. The half reaction time for the process of the alactic oxygen debt payment is correspondingly decreased to $\ln(2/1 \cdot 87) = 0 \cdot 37$ min or 22 s. This last value is therefore the correct one for the rate of phosphagen resynthesis by reaction b in the scheme of Fig. 1.4.

The calculation of the oxygen spent for the delayed work of the heart and respiratory muscles is more difficult, but it does not appreciably affect the conclusions outlined above. In fact the increased ventilation in recovery to pay a 2-l oxygen debt is probably 40 l, at an average rate of 30 l min^{-1}: this involves an oxygen consumption of only about 5 ml (Milic-Emili and Petit 1960; Margaria, Milic-Emili, Petit, and Cavagna 1960). The increased circulation in recovery is probably about 15 l, and the extra cost of this may be about 40–50 ml of oxygen.

The relationship between oxygen debt and oxygen consumption has been investigated on the isolated mammalian muscle by di Prampero and Piiper (1966). Here also a linear relationship was found between the two parameters. The slope of the line corresponds to a half reaction time for this process of 17 s, i.e. a value not appreciably different from that obtained above from experiments in man under more physiological conditions as calculated from the data of Margaria *et al.* 1933, and from those obtained by di Prampero and Margaria (1968, 1969).

Summary concerning the exergonic processes in muscle

The *power* and the *capacity* of the exergonic processes taking place in muscle, expressed as oxidative energy required, together with the time-course of the oxygen debt contraction and payment for average young normal subjects are given in Table 1.1. Data from single individuals may differ appreciably from the average values given in the table: they are very indicative of the performance possibilities of a subject and they should be known for every single individual, when required in such area of activity as in work or in sport physiology.

The most important factors are: (a) the maximum power of the oxidative mechanism and (b) the maximum power of the alactic mechanism; the second is also the maximum power of which an individual is capable. These two factors provide satisfactory information on the capacity for performing work and for contracting an oxygen debt.

Of the other data indicated in the table, the *speed of payment of the oxygen debt* is presumably the same for all subjects, for it depends mainly on the chemical enzymatic composition of the muscle and on the oxygen supply. The *time for full contraction of the oxygen debt*, on the other hand, depends on the capability of the subject and on his will to perform at a maximal level: it also depends on the capacity and the power of his anaerobic mechanisms.

The *capacity of the alactic mechanism* is related mainly to the muscular masses; it is not likely that the chemical composition of

Table 1.1
Capacity and power of exergonic mechanisms in muscular contraction (maximal exercise)

	Power	Capacity	Maximum	Oxygen debt Minimum time for a full contraction	(half reaction time)
	(kcal per kg h^{-1})	(cal per kg)	(ml per kg)	(sec)	(min)
Alactacid mechanism	48	100 (200)†	20 (40)†	8	0·5
Oxidative mechanism	13	∞	—	—	—
Lactacid mechanism	25	250	52	40	15

† Values in brackets are for supramaximal exercise.

the muscle can change appreciably. Training, which involves an increase of the muscular masses, should therefore increase correspondingly the capacity and also obviously the power of the alactic mechanism.

The *capacity and the power of the lactacid mechanism* depend not only on the muscle masses of the subject but also on his nutritional state, and more specifically on the glycogen content of the muscles. This changes from time to time and it cannot be considered a constant characteristic of the subject.

It is obviously important that an individual participating in a challenge test, such as a sporting competition, should be in a good state of nutrition, at least so far as the glycogen stores in the muscles are concerned. This can be achieved by a prevailing carbohydrate diet, particularly in the two or three days preceding the performance. The glycogen content of the muscles can then increase from an average 1·5 g per 100 g on a normal mixed diet to 2·5 g per 100 g of muscle. It has been claimed by Saltin and Hermansen (1967) that the glycogen content can be increased to 4 or 5 g per 100 g of muscle if the two days of intense carbohydrate diet are preceded by the depletion of carbohydrate stores in muscles, obtained either by prolonged exercise to exhaustion or by adopting an exclusively protein and fat diet for a couple of days.

The measurement of the maximum muscular power

The direct measurement of the maximum aerobic and anaerobic muscular power as described above is technically difficult and time-consuming. Simpler methods have therefore been devised that avoid stressing the subjects and do not require special knowledge or skill on the part of the operator. These methods can be used by non-physiologists such as physical educators, or technicians.

Maximum anaerobic power

The maximum muscular power due to the anaerobic (alactic) mechanism in man can be estimated simply by measuring the maximum work that can be performed within 3–5 s, namely before the intervention of oxidative and glycolytic mechanisms, as indicated by the data in Fig. 1.14.

When climbing stairs two steps at a time at top speed, after a short initial phase of acceleration which lasts no longer than 2 s, the speed of progression reaches a constant value until 4–5 s have elapsed, after which it decreases progressively (Fig. 1.18). In this constant-speed phase the external work performed consists almost exclusively in lifting the body, for the work involved in the acceleration and deceleration at each step is negligible. The phase of initial acceleration can be overcome by a 2-m run on the flat before initiating the stair climbing.

The steps should be about 175 mm high (2 steps = 350 mm). The time required to run an even number of steps should be measured with an electronic watch accurate to 1/100 s.

The vertical component of the speed v_V can then be calculated and expressed in metres per second. The same figure will also give a measure of the mechanical energy W_V expressed in kg m per kg of body weight per second. This amounts to about 1·4 kg m per kg s^{-1} for young fit subjects of 20 to 30 years of age, decreasing with age to about half that value at 70 years. Scattering of the individual data is however very high, which allows a selection of the most fit subjects (Fig. 1.19).

By dividing the mechanical power so obtained by the efficiency,

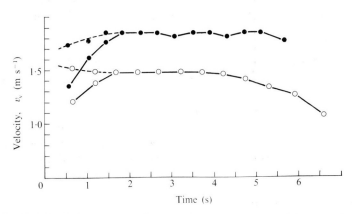

Fig. 1.18. Vertical component of the speed in metres per second in two subjects (open and closed circles) running at top speed up a staircase two steps at a time, the height of the two steps combined being 35 cm and their horizontal width 65 cm. On the abscissa, time after running started. To the early values obtained during the acceleration phase, the work necessary to increase the velocity in the direction of progression has been calculated and the corresponding equivalent increase in vertical speed added (broken line) (from Margaria, Aghemo, and Rovelli 1966.)

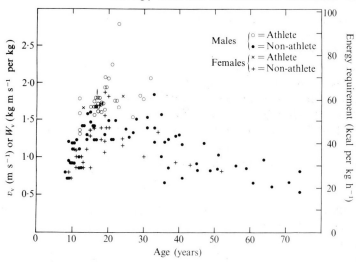

Fig. 1.19. Vertical component of the speed (m s^{-1}), or maximal anaerobic power (kg m per kg s^{-1}) as a function of age in 131 subjects running at top speed up on staircase. Those regularly active in sport (athletes) give generally higher values. A value of 25 per cent for the mechanical efficiency of the exercise has been assumed to calculate the energy requirement in kcal per kg h^{-1} from mechanical power output. (From Margaria *et al.* 1966.)

which appears to be 0·25 for exercise of this kind (Margaria *et al.* 1963*a*) the power expressed in oxidative energy requirement is obtained. This appears to be 3–4 times greater than the maximum aerobic power: it amounts to 750 cal per kilogram of body weight and per minute, corresponding to an oxygen requirement of 150 ml per kg min^{-1}.

This test is simple enough; it requires little time to carry out, and it is well accepted by subjects because it is short enough not to lead to exhaustion. It can therefore be used on a wide scale, for example in population studies (Fig. 1.19). It has, however, the limitation of measuring only the muscular power of the lower limbs, a fact that must be taken into consideration when assessing the work capacity of individuals engaged in working mainly with their arms.

The maximum aerobic power

This is the expression of the maximum rate of reaction *c* of the scheme of Fig. 1.4, namely of oxidation. It can be measured directly through the maximum oxygen consumption by performing supramaximal exercise that leads to exhaustion in 6–10 min, and by measuring the oxygen consumption in the last 2 min of the performance. In more strenuous exercises leading to exhaustion in less than 6 min the oxygen consumption measured at the end of the run is higher than in a more prolonged run, as shown in Fig. 1.20 (Brambilla and Cerretelli 1958).

More feasible and probably just as accurate is the indirect method, which is based on the linearity of the relationship between oxygen consumption and heart rate per minute f:

$$f = x - y\dot{V}_{O_2} \tag{1.8}$$

By determining the heart rate during exercise by means of an electrocardiograph at two values of oxygen consumption, the constants x and y can be determined and eqn (1.8) defined: if the maximum heart rate (f^{max}) is known, the maximal oxygen consumption can then be easily calculated. Asmussen *et al.* (1957) and Astrand and Riming (1954) give one of the constants x or y a predetermined value, and the heart rate taken at one level only of $\dot{V}_{O_2}$ is used to calculate the other constant: with this procedure they obtain data that they claim are reliable within ± 10 per cent.

This method can be improved by making at least two, or better

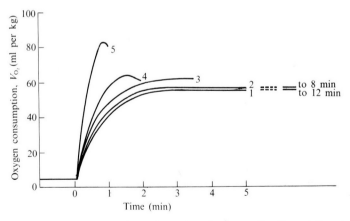

Fig. 1.20. Oxygen consumption ml per kg min^{-1} as a function of time in 5 supramaximal exercises at different intensities leading to exhaustion at the time indicated at the end of each curve (average of 'normal' subjects). (From Brambilla and Cerretelli 1958.)

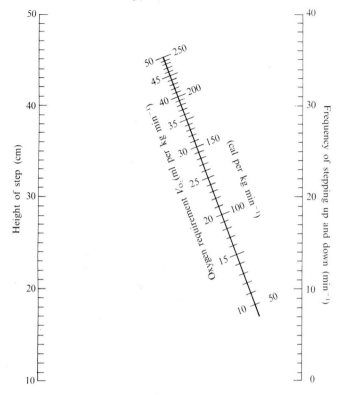

Fig. 1.21. Nomogram for the rapid calculation of the energy expenditure in the stepping exercise, expressed in calorie equivalent or volume of oxygen (assuming 1 ml O_2 equivalent to 5 cal) per kilogram of body weight and per minute, when the height of the step and the frequency of stepping are known. (From Margaria, Aghemo, and Rovelli 1965.)

four, determinations of f at different $\dot{V}_{O_2}$ values. If the energy cost of an exercise is exactly known, as in stepping up to and down from a bench of a given height at a given frequency (Rovelli and Aghemo 1963), one can avoid the determination of $\dot{V}_{O_2}$ and limit the analysis to the recording of the heart rate during the fourth to the fifth minute of the exercise, when a steady heart rate is reached.

The energy cost of stepping up and down has been found to be effectively constant for all fit individuals. The data are summarized in the nomogram of Fig. 1.21 (Margaria *et al.* 1965).

By measuring the heart rates f_1 and f_2 at two work-loads at oxygen consumptions of $\dot{V}'_{O_2}$ and $\dot{V}''_{2O_2}$ respectively, the maximal heart rate f^{max} being known, the maximal oxygen consumption can be calculated as from eqn (1.8) by the equation

$$\dot{V}^{max}_{O_2} = \frac{f^{max}(\dot{V}''_{O_2} - \dot{V}'_{O_2}) + f''(\dot{V}'_{O_2} - f\dot{V}''_{O_2})}{f'' - f'}. \tag{1.9}$$

For routine tests on fit adults stepping on a 40-cm bench at a frequency of 15 and 25 times per minute has been found convenient. These work-rates correspond to $\dot{V}_{O_2}$ values of 22.0 ml per kg min^{-1} and 32·4 ml per kg min^{-1} respectively. To avoid lengthy calculations the nomogram of Fig. 1.22 can be used and the maximum oxygen consumption per kilogram of body weight and per minute can be read directly on the appropriate line corresponding to maximum heart rates of 160, 180, or 200 beats per minute.

For children and for old people or for unfit subjects a 30-cm step may be preferable. For this the nomogram of Fig. 1.23 has been constructed on the same principle as that of Fig. 1.22, the two exercises consisting of stepping on and off the 30-cm bench 15 and 27 times per minute respectively.

The maximum heart-rate value can be assessed by having the subject perform supramaximal exercise. This, however, is not constant during the exercise; it may therefore be preferable to assume a given value according to the age of the subject. The data from different authors assembled in Fig. 1.22 indicate how the maximum heart rate decreases with age.

If two sets of exercise on the 40-cm and on the 30-cm bench are made, four experimental points will define the linear relation connecting heart rate with oxygen consumption and the data on maximum aerobic power will be more reliable.

Stepping up and down a bench has been selected for this purpose as the best ergometric procedure. It has several advantages over other procedures and particularly over the widely used bicycle ergometer: (1) a step can be found anywhere; (2) it is unexpensive; (3) it does not require calibration, except the exact measure of its height; (4) the exercise is much more familiar than cycling; (5) the bicycle is generally ill adjusted to all subjects, even those who are accustomed to cycling; (6) the energy expenditure is proportional to the body lift and within reasonable limits

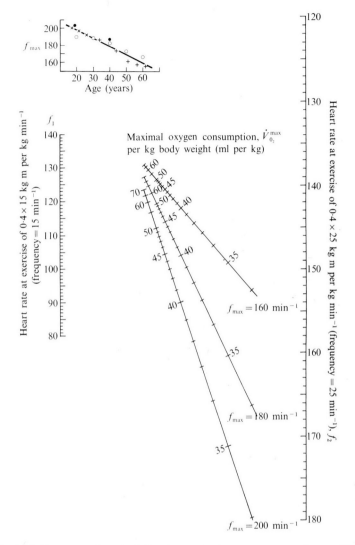

Fig. 1.22. Nomogram for calculating the maximal oxygen consumption per kilogram of body weight and per minute when the heart rate is at steady state, in the two intensities of exercise as indicated (stepping up and down a bench 40 cm high at 15 min^{-1} and 25 min^{-1}), are known (from Margaria *et al.* 1965). At the top the maximum heart rate f_{max} is plotted as a function of age (data from different authors), to give the appropriate values used below ($f_{max} = 200$, 180, or 160 min^{-1}) when the subject's age is known.

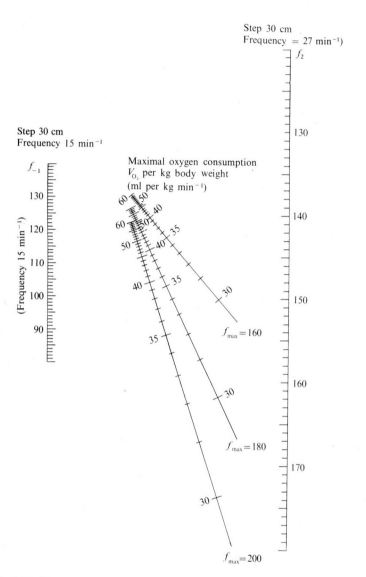

Fig. 1.23. Nomogram to calculate maximum oxygen consumption from heart rate values when stepping up and down a bench 30 cm high, at frequencies of 15 min⁻¹ (f_1) and 27 min⁻¹ (f_2). (From Margaria *et al.* 1965.)

is independent of the height of the step and of the step frequency; the cost of the exercise per unit of body weight is constant for normal subjects and independent of age, sex, body size, etc.; in other words, the efficiency of this exercise, unlike those, such as cycling, that require a certain skill, is the same for all fit subjects. The test is therefore valid for whole populations.

The exercise is performed with the subject holding a firm handle with one hand: this gives more confidence to the subject during the exercise, without altering significantly the energy requirement. Care should be taken that the exercise is performed properly, and particularly (a) that full lift of the body takes place in the 'up' phase of the stepping, with full extension of the knees, (b) that the subject follows exactly the frequency of the stepping, as dictated by the metronome, and (c) that the lift phase is made with both the right and the left leg alternatively.

This test is well accepted by the subjects, for it does not require any particular skill, it needs very little training, and does not lead to exhaustion.

A simple relationship between maximum aerobic power and performance in running

It is well established that in running the net cost of speed maintenance per kilogram of body weight and per metre covered is a constant, independent of speed, at least up to the maximum speed values at which a steady-state condition can be attained (see pp. 73–4) (Margaria *et al.* 1963*a*). This cos amounts to about 0.9 cal m^{-1} per kg when running on the level on a treadmill, or to roughly 1 cal per kg m^{-1} or 0.2 ml of oxygen per kilogram per metre when running on the road, allowance being made for wind resistance, inequalities of the ground, etc.

Assuming that $\dot{V}_{O_2}$ not involved in the process of running amounts to 6 ml per kg min^{-1}, a figure slightly higher than the rest pre-exercise value, the maximal distance m covered in the time t at the expense of oxidation only is

$$m = 5(\dot{V}_{O_2}^{max} - 6)t, \qquad (1.10)$$

where $\dot{V}_{O_2}^{max}$ is the maximum oxygen consumption of the subject.

When running a given distance at top speed the energy from glycolysis must also be taken into account, besides that due to oxidation: this is equivalent to about the maximal oxygen consumption in 1 minute (p. 20). By adding this factor, eqn (1.10) can then be corrected to

$$m = 5(\dot{V}_{O_2}^{max} - 6)t + 5\dot{V}_{O_2}^{max}. \tag{1.11}$$

At the onset of the exercise phosphagen cleavage is an important source of energy. This, however, in a not too strenuous exercise that can be maintained for at least 2 minutes, is about equivalent to the $\dot{V}_{O_2}$ deficit (contraction of the alactic oxygen debt): it may therefore be assumed that the total energy from these two sources at the onset of the exercise is the same as the maximum energy from steady-state oxidations. Eqn (1.11) is then representative of the conditions met in running at maximum speed a distance not less than 1000 m. If the maximum aerobic power $\dot{V}_{O_2}^{max}$ of a subject is known, the minimum time necessary to cover a given distance m can therefore be calculated (from eqn (1.11)). As for any given t value the distance covered m is a linear function of $\dot{V}_{O_2}^{max}$, a nomogram can be constructed relating these three variables (Fig. 1.24). It is then easy to predict the maximum oxygen consumption required per minute to cover the distance m in a given time t, or the time required to cover a given distance m when $\dot{V}_{O_2}^{max}$ is known.

For example, it appears from Fig. 1.24 that a subject with a maximum aerobic power of 50 ml per kg min^{-1} of oxygen will not be able to cover 10 000 m in less than 44 min. On the other hand, to cover 10 000 m in less than 28 min 3 s, 5000 m in less than 13 min 29 s, or 1500 m in less than 3 min 37 s (world records in 1969), $\dot{V}_{O_2}^{max}$ must be not less than 74, 75, or 70 ml per kg min^{-1} respectively.

The values obtained from Fig. 1.24 are only approximate, for no allowance has been made for differences in the efficiency of running of different subjects, for their state of nutrition and their capacity for producing lactic acid from glycogen, for differences in the track or the pavement, for wind resistance, for the capacity of the subject to maintain his maximum oxygen consumption for the whole time of the performance, etc.

Eqn (1.11) and Fig. 1.24 do not apply for distances shorter than 1000 m, for the assumptions made above are not then valid. In fact, in very short sprints at top speed the energy derived from phosphagen cleavage at the onset of the exercise may greatly

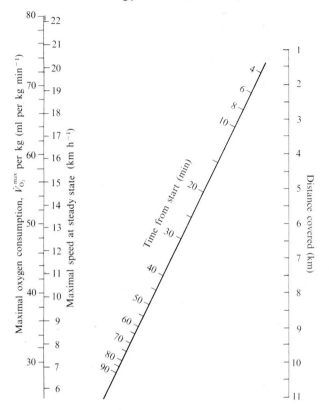

Fig. 1.24. Nomogram to relate the maximum aerobic power $\dot{V}_{O_2}^{max}$ of the subject with the minimum time necessary in minutes, when running at maximum speed to cover the distance in kilometres according to eqn (1.11). The corresponding maintainance speed of running at the expense of oxidations only, as from eqn (1.10), is also indicated on the left-hand vertical line.

exceed the oxygen deficit, and the work involved in acceleration at the start and in meeting wind resistance, which can be neglected in a middle- or long-distance run (being only a small fraction of the total work performed), may be appreciable. Eqn (1.11) and Fig. 1.24 are valid only for running, not for walking, where the cost per metre covered is very different and is not independent of speed. Their validity is, however, not limited to athletes, but extends to the whole population, including women, the elderly, and children, since the energy cost of running, when referred to the distance covered and to body weight, is virtually the same for all fit people.

In spite of its limitations Fig. 1.24 can give indications that may be of practical value both in sport and in recreation. Conversely it can also be used to assess the maximum aerobic power $V_{O_2}^{max}$ of a subject when the distance covered and the time taken in a running event of duration greater than about 5 min are known. This is particularly useful, for many popular tests common in athletics consist of measuring the time employed to run a given distance: the athletic capacity of the subject is then given in empirical units called 'scores', rather than in the more rational unit of 'power', which should in my opinion be generally adopted, not only by physiologists, but also by physical educators, trainers, and athletes.

Intermittent strenuous exercise

Of the two mechanisms of anaerobic energy expenditure, phosphagen cleavage and glycolysis, the first has many advantages over the second: the alactic mechanism can develop a much higher power; the payment of the oxygen debt is very fast; and phosphagen cleavage does not involve any alteration of the acid–base equilibrium of the body fluids. The lactacid mechanism, on the other hand, though it has a somewhat greater capacity, has less power than the alactic; the payment of the lactacid debt is slow, being still incomplete after an hour of recovery; and, in particular the lactic acid induces a state of acidosis characterized by clear objective and subjective symptoms including, among other things, a decreased performance and a strong sensation of discomfort.

Whenever possible, therefore, the convenience of limiting the contraction of an oxygen debt to the alactic fraction, without incurring a lactacid debt, is evident. This is made possible because, as is shown by the experiments summarized in Fig. 1.12, lactic acid formation does not begin until the alactic mechanism is near exhaustion. The two processes are quite distinctly separated in time, even in the most strenuous exercise.

This being the case, if a period of supramaximal exercise does not last long enough to reach the lactacid phase, lactic acid production does not begin, and only an alactic oxygen debt is contracted: if time is then allowed for this alactic oxygen debt to

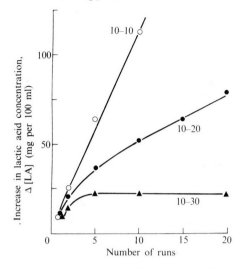

Fig. 1.25. The concentration of lactic acid in the blood is shown as a function of the number of running cycles on a treadmill (18 km h^{-1} at an incline of 15 per cent); the cycle consisted in 10-s run followed by rest of respectively 10, 20, and 30 s, as indicated (from Margaria *et al.* 1969.)

be paid, the exercise can be resumed very soon after, for the same time as before, and cycles of work and rest can be repeated indefinitely.

Fig. 1.25 shows the results of some experiments devised to test the validity of the hypothesis that supramaximal exercise, if performed intermittently, can be made to last a long time, giving a very high total work performance (Margaria, Oliva, di Prampero, and Cerretelli 1969). A subject ran on an inclined treadmill at such a speed as to lead to exhaustion in about 35 s. In one series of tests the run lasted only 10 s; 10 s rest was then allowed, after which the exercise was resumed. Ten successive runs could be made under these conditions, 100 s of exercise altogether; the lactic acid concentration in the blood reached a maximum value of 1·25 g l^{-1} at the end of the tenth run.

If the rest period between the 10 s of exercise was 20 s, the subject could perform 20 runs, totalling 200 s of exercise; the lactic acid in the blood increased at a much slower rate, reaching a maximum value of 0·6 g/l^{-1} at the end of the twentieth run.

If the rest period was 30 s the lactic acid in the blood, did not increase any further after the first few runs, in which a concentration of 0.20 g l^{-1} was reached, and the exercise could be carried on for many hours.

The slight initial increase in the blood lactic acid is due to the sluggishness of the oxidative mechanism and thence to the relatively anaerobic condition of the limb muscles at the beginning of exercise. This particular condition is also evident when the work intensity is submaximal, as mentioned above (see Fig. 1.11).

The capacity for strenuous supramaximal work can thus be increased substantially if the work is made intermittent. This principle may find application whenever strenuous work is to be done (see also Edwards, Ekclund, Harris, Hesser, Hultman, Melcheor, and Wigertz 1973). For example, if an athlete training for the 400 m covers the whole distance at the maximum speed, he will incur a state of acidosis that will be removed only after a rest of at least $1\frac{1}{2}$ h. In a total of 4 h, he can therefore run at most three stretches, covering a total distance of 1200 m. If he runs instead short stretches of only 100 m at the same speed, allowing intervals of 30 s between them, he will not incur any lactic acid production. In 4 h he can perform 360 cycles, covering a total distance of 36 000 m. He will thus perform 30 times as much work as he could have done had the exercise been continuous.

Delayed production of lactic acid

As mentioned earlier, to obtain a sample that is representative of the total lactic acid formed in the body, the blood must be drawn during recovery after enough time has elapsed to allow for the diffusion and uniform distribution of lactic acid into the body fluids. It is not, however, possible to discriminate between the lactic acid produced during the exercise and possibly produced afterwards, early in recovery.

In calculating the data for Table 1.1 and Figs 1.12 and 1.15 it was assumed that all lactic acid was produced during exercise. These data refer therefore to the final balance, and are not representative of the course of the various chemical and energetic processes that actually take place during exercise or recovery.

That some lactic acid is produced in the early period of recovery after exercise appears obvious if one considers that the mechanical events in muscular contraction must coincide with the cleavage of ATP and phosphagen. The reactions related to lactic

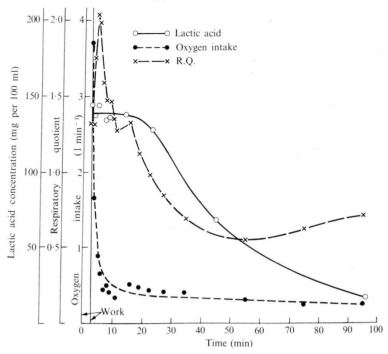

Fig. 1.26. Oxygen intake, lactic acid concentration, and respiratory quotient in a subject after a rum on the treadmill at a speed of 14 km h^{-1} for 3 min to exhaustion (from Margaria, Edwards, and Dill 1933).

acid formation and to oxidation must follow. When exercise is suddenly stopped these must still be active early in recovery.

Evidence for the delayed lactic acid production in isolated muscle was given by Embden in 1925. Further evidence is provided by the anaerobic recovery of isolated frog muscle as described above (see Fig. 1.17). In man delayed lactic acid production is indicated by the very high respiratory quotient R.Q. that is found early in recovery particularly after strenuous exercise, in which values as high as 2·00 have been found (Fig. 1.26). The high carbon dioxide output leading to such an increase of the respiratory quotient may not necessarily be due to actual lactic acid production in that period, but simply to delayed diffusion into the blood of lactic acid accumulated within the muscle cells. In view of the considerations set out above, however, delayed formation of lactic acid must take place in man after exhausting exercise. At the end of very exhausting exercise the muscle phosphagen is practically completely split and some time is necessary for it to resynthesize in order to reach a threshold level at which no lactic acid production takes place and further resynthesis is supported only by the energy provided by oxidations (see p. 26).

Di Prampero and Margaria (1973), using an indirect method, measured the delayed lactic acid production in short bursts of maximal exercise that could be maintained for only a few seconds. They found that at the higher work-load leading to exhaustion in 10 s the delayed lactic acid amounted to about two-thirds of the total produced as an effect of the exercise. In less strenuous exercise, leading to exhaustion in 40 s, practically all the lactic acid is actually produced during the exercise; this time appears to be long enough for lactic acid to attain the maximum concentration in the blood. At the end of such long-sustained exercise the glycolytic mechanism presumably is exhausted, and when the exercise comes to a stop no further formation of lactic acid takes place, even if the phosphagen level in the muscle is below the critical threshold at which the glycolytic mechanism is triggered.

The course of the contraction and payment of the oxygen debt in supramaximal exercise

The oxygen debt is generally measured from the curve of the extra oxygen consumption (above the rest value) in the early phase of recovery after exercise. The area delimited by this curve and the coordinate, corrected for the extra rest oxygen consumption, is representative of the oxygen debt (Fig. 1.27): it amounts to about 20 ml. In supramaximal exercise probably all the phosphagen is split during activity, corresponding to the contraction of an oxygen debt of 40 ml (see Fig. 1.27): only part of it, 30 ml, is resynthesized directly by oxidation at the end of the exercise: the remaining 10 ml is resynthesized indirectly through the contraction of a lactacid debt (Fig. 1.28).

A rough but fairly accurate picture of the events that take place in exercise during the active and recovery periods can therefore be sketched. At the onset of *maximal exercise* the

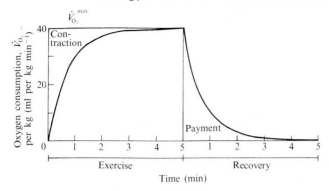

Fig. 1.27. Oxygen consumption at the onset of a maximal exercise, corresponding to an oxygen consumption of 40 ml per kilogram of body weight per minute, and during recovery. Areas indicated 'contraction' and 'payment', refer to the alactic oxygen debt.

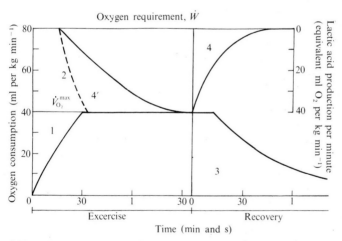

Fig. 1.28. When the oxygen requirement increases to twice the maximum oxygen consumption, 80 ml per kg min^{-1}, the oxygen consumption rate increases twice as rapidly, to reach the 40 ml level, which is maintained for the whole duration of the performance. The contraction of the alactic debt is now indicated by areas 1, 2, and 4'. Area 4, a fraction of the total area due to lactic acid, indicates the delayed lactic acid production which is used to pay the amount of alactic debt indicated as 4'. Area 3 corresponds to the payment of the alactic debt represented by areas 1 and 2. The ordinate at the right is the lactic acid production per min expressed as equivalent oxygen consumption.

consumption of oxygen increases exponentially to reach the maximum value (40 ml per kg min^{-1}), as shown in Fig. 1.26. At the end of the exercise the oxygen consumption decreases exponentially to the rest value. Under these conditions no appreciable amount of lactic acid is formed (see p. 3), and the oxygen dept is only alactic.

In *supramaximal exercise*, with an energy requirement twice as great (80 ml min^{-1}), the oxygen consumption at the onset of the exercise increases twice as fast, to reach the $\dot{V}_{O_2}^{max}$ value in a shorter time, as shown in Fig. 1.28. At the beginning of the exercise the energy requirement is met substantially by phosphagen cleavage, which leads to the contraction of an alactic debt. Lactic acid formation is initiated only later, when a noticeable quantity of the total muscle phosphagen, about 50 per cent, is split, and approaches a steady level of formation within a few seconds. When this level is reached the production of lactic acid is the only mechanism responsible for the supramaximal quota of the energy requirement. The lactic acid formation mechanism seems to be triggered by the (anaerobic) quota of 50 per cent split phosphagen.

During recovery after supramaximal exercise the oxygen consumption does not drop suddenly, as after maximal exercise, but it maintains the maximum level for 10–15 s until the concentration of split phosphagen in the muscles is reduced to a lower value, presumably about 50 per cent of the total phosphagen; it then decreases exponentially with the same kinetics as after an aerobic exercise. In the early period of recovery neither is lactic acid formation stopped. This is due to the persistence of anaerobic conditions in the muscle cells, and a fraction of the total lactic acid is formed to aid the resynthesis of the phosphagen split: this fraction of the phosphagen resynthesis, which does not take place at the expense of the oxidation, does not appear as an alactic debt as measured conventionally from the area of the oxygen consumption curve after exercise: it may be estimated at about 10 ml of oxygen.

In conclusion, only half the phosphagen content of the muscle is split during maximal steady-state aerobic exercise and this is all resynthesized in recovery by oxidation. In strenuous supramaximal exercise to exhaustion the remaining half is also presumably split by the end of the exercise; of this second half, about equal amounts are resynthesized during recovery by energy from oxidation, and by energy from delayed lactic acid formation.

A hydraulic model of the energetic processes in muscle

A hydraulic model of the energy sources in muscular exercise is given in Fig. 1.29. The fluid in vessel GP (representing *phosphagen*) is directly connected with the outside through the tap T which regulates the flow (*energy expenditure*): when this is closed (rest) the upper level of fluid in GP is the same as in the communicating vessel O_2 which is of infinite capacity, corresponding to the *source of oxidative energy*.

The tap T regulates the outflow (energy expenditure or phosphagen breakdown), which results in a fall in the level of the fluid in GP. Because of the higher level of the fluid in the vessel O_2, fluid from this flows to GP through the communicating tube R_1, which offers a greater resistance than that offered by tap T. If the flow through T is not too great, the level in GP will be lower than at rest, reaching an equilibrium value as fluid flows continuously from the vessel O_2 through R_1. The flow through R_1 (corresponding to the *oxygen consumption*, $\dot{V}_{O_2}$) depends on the pressure gradient between the two compartments, which in turn depends on the flow through tap T.

When the opening of T is such as to allow a flow higher than

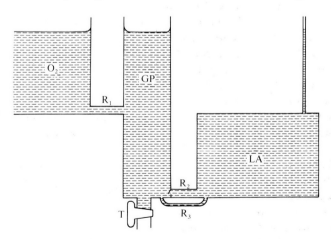

Fig. 1.29. A hydraulic model of energy sources in muscular activity. For explanation see text.

the flow through R_1 (i.e. when the energy expenditure is higher than the oxygen consumption, supramaximal exercise) the level in GP falls below R_1. The flow of liquid from O_2 to GP then reaches a constant maximum value, independent of the level in GP, and defined only by the height of the fluid in O_2 and by the resistance of R_1 (*maximum oxygen consumption*). The flow through R_1 is then insufficient to maintain a steady level of the fluid in GP, and the vessel GP will tend to be emptied.

A decrease of the level of the fluid in GP below R_1 causes fluid to flow from the vessel LA to GP (*lactic acid formation*) according to the different level of the fluid in the two compartments, and to the resistance of the communicating channel R_2: this is provided with a one-way valve allowing flow from LA to GP but not vice versa.

Because of this additional flow of fluid, a steady level of the fluid in vessel GP below the opening R_1 can be maintained if the flow of the fluid through T is not too high, but only for a limited time, owing to the limited capacity of vessel LA. The resistance of tube R_2, though lower than the resistance of R_1 is higher than the resistance of tap T when fully open, so that maximum flow through T cannot be maintained even when a considerable amount of fluid is contained in the vessel LA. The flow through R_2 represents the *power of the lactacid mechanism*.

If when the vessel GP is nearly empty the tap T is suddenly shut, the vessel GP is refilled (*recovery*) through the channel R_1. At first it fills at a constant speed (*constant oxygen consumption*, see Fig. 1.27); later, when the level of the fluid in GP has reached the height of R_1, at a progressively reduced speed following an exponential function, until the level in GP is the same as in O_2 (*payment of the alactic oxygen debt*).

Suppose now that the tap T is closed before the vessel LA is completely emptied and the level in LA is higher than in GP. In the first phase of recovery some fluid will also flow from LA to GP until the level in GP equals the level in LA; this corresponds to the *delayed lactic acid formation*, representing payment of a fraction of the alactic debt by contracting a lactacid debt. Under these conditions GP is refilled very rapidly because two factors are at work at the same time.

The vessel LA is also refilled when the tap T is closed (*payment of the lactacid oxygen debt*); but the rate of refilling is very slow, since it takes place through the very resistant communication R_3 short-circuiting the communication R_2.

The extension of the vessel LA, a narrow tube, represents the *lactic acid content in the blood at rest*: this does not contribute appreciably to the flow through T.

The efficiency of the processes involved in energy transformation

As it is well known, the combustion of 1 glucose unit of glycogen through the glycolytic reaction and the Krebs cycle leads to the synthesis of 39 mol high-energy phosphate (phosphagen). As 6 mol or 12 gram-atoms of oxygen are necessary to burn 1 mol of glucose, the ratio of phosphate to oxygen P/O for this process is $39/12 = 3.25$.

One mole of glucose yields 675 000 cal, while 39 mol phosphagen, assigning to this the same energy yield of creatine phosphate, 11 000 cal mol^{-1} (Wilkie 1968), corresponds to 429 000 cal. The *efficiency of the oxidative synthesis of phosphagen* amounts therefore to $429\,000/675\,000 = 0.635$.

The *overall mechanical efficiency in aerobic muscular exercise* is 0.25 (see p. 74). As this is the resultant of the product of the efficiencies of the two component processes, the production of mechanical energy from phosphagen cleavage and the oxidative synthesis of phosphagen, the efficiency of the *production of mechanical work from phosphagen cleavage* must therefore be: $0.25/0.635 = 0.40$.

It is also well known that in the glycolytic process 3 mol phosphagen (33 000 cal) are synthesized for every glucose unit converted to lactic acid; the energy yield of the glycolysis corresponds to 43 200 cal per glucose unit, according to a calorific equivalent of 240 cal per g of lactic acid, as found experimentally (p. 00). *The efficiency of the synthesis of phosphagen* from glycolysis appears therefore to be appreciably higher than for oxidation, i.e. $33\,000/43\,200 = 0.76$.

The resynthesis of lactic acid to glycogen, however, involving the synthesis of 3 mol phosphagen, requires 33 000 cal per glucose unit. Let us assume that 1 mol lactic acid (or glucose equivalent) is oxidized while 9 mol are resynthesized to glycogen, i.e. that the combustion coefficient of lactic acid is 1/10 (see p.

5). The *efficiency* of this can be calculated as $9 \times$ 33 000/429 000 = 0·70. The *overall mechanical efficiency of muscular exercise performed anaerobically at the expenses of glycolysis* would then be $0·76 \times 0·70 = 0·215$, not much lower than in aerobic exercise.

Energy equivalent of phosphagen cleavage and lactic acid formation

From the efficiency value of phosphagen resynthesis from oxidation it can be calculated that 1 mol *phosphagen breakdown* corresponds to an *overall energy requirement* of 11 000/0·635 = 17 300 cal. Since the energy equivalent of lactic acid is 240 cal g^{-1}, 1 mol lactic acid corresponds to $90 \times 240 = 21 600$ cal. The ratio is then

$$\frac{\text{cal per mol phosphagen}}{\text{cal per mol lactic acid}} = 0·8.$$

For a given energy expenditure supplied by phosphagen cleavage alone $1/0·8 = 1·25$ mol phosphagen would therefore be required, while were lactic acid the only source of energy only one mol of this substance should be produced.

Experiments performed on isolated dog gastrocnemius (Cerretelli *et al.* 1969; Piiper, di Prampero, and Cerretelli 1968; di Prampero and Margaria 1969) confirm these data.

More recent confirmation has come from an elegant experiment performed by Jones (1973) on mammalian muscle, in which the sequence in which the energy sources come into play in muscular activity, as outlined above, was quantitatively described.

An isolated mouse gastrocnemius was stimulated tetanically for 45 s and the concentrations of ATP, phosphocreatine, and lactate were measured at intervals in the muscle itself (Fig. 1.30).

The ATP did not change appreciably in the whole course of the tetanus. In the first 15 s only CP was split, while the concentration of lactate was about constant. From the data (Fig. 1.29) the rate of cleavage of CP can be calculated as amounting to 0·094 μmol s^{-1} per gram of dry muscle, and per gram of tension developed. In the last 20 s of contraction CP and ATP were practically constant: only lactic acid increased in concentration in muscular tissue, and this took place at a rate of 0·066 μmol s^{-1} per gram of muscle and per gram of tension.

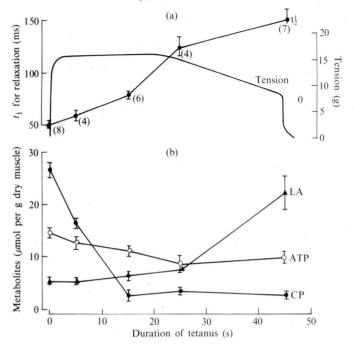

Fig. 1.30. Concentration of lactic acid, ATP, and CP in an isolated mouse gastrcnemius in the course of a 45-s tetanic contraction (b). (a) The tension developed during the whole tetanus and the relaxation time (which increases with fatigue). (From Jones 1973.)

The ratio of the rate of cleavage of CP, in the initial phase of the contraction, to the lactic acid formation rate towards the end of the tetanus is then 1·4; in other words, 1 mol lactic acid is equivalent to the splitting of 1·4 mol CP. This is in fairly good agreement with the fact that a smaller amount of energy is obtained from the cleavage of 1 mol phosphagen than from the formation of 1 mol of lactic acid from glycogen, as calculated above.

Jones's experiment, besides showing clearly that the lactic acid source of energy comes into play after the phosphagen cleavage mechanism is about exhausted, or at least well advanced, therefore confirms the quantitative data for the energy obtained from the two anaerobic mechanisms and for their mechanical efficiency, as discussed above. It also appears from Fig. 1.29 that lactic acid formation sets in when the concentration of unsplit phosphagen (ATP+CP) in muscle drops to about half the rest value. This supports the suggestion made above that a drop of that magnitude is the *triggering mechanism* that brings glycolysis into play in muscular activity.

Conclusion

The chemical and energy transformations that take place in muscle were still rather obscure only a few years ago, but now appear sufficiently clear to provide evidence, at least in a general way, of the means by which men and animals can perform mechanical work. With this knowledge it is possible to rationalize exercise in order to obtain greater mechanical power and the maximum amount of work in a given time, or a higher efficiency with great energy saving. Wide application of this knowledge is desirable, not only in sports and in athletics, but also in ergonomics, in order to increase the productive capacity, the comfort, and the health of those whose occupations call for the performance of substantial amounts of mechanical work and high energy expenditure.

2 Some fundamental cardiorespiratory functional changes met in exercise and other conditions

THE MAXIMUM oxygen intake is an integrative characteristic that depends among others on several circulatory and respiratory functions, some of which are very significant and some of great interest. They may be calculated from the maximum oxygen intake as determined by the method outlined in Chapter 1 if a few additional observations or some reasonable assumptions are made.

The oxygen consumption can be calculated from circulatory data according to Fick's equation:

$$\dot{V}_{O_2} = \dot{Q}([O_2]_a - [O_2]_{\bar{v}}).\dagger \qquad (2.1)$$

† The following symbols are used in this chapter.

$[Hb]_{tot}$: the oxygen capacity of the blood (litres of oxygen per litre of blood)

$[HbO_2]$: concentration of oxygen bound with haemoglobin in litres per litre of blood

$[O_2]_{diss}$: concentration of physically dissolved oxygen, in litres per litre of blood

$[O_2] = [HbO_2] + [O_2]_{diss}$: concentration of oxygen in litres per litre of blood

$S = \dfrac{[HbO_2]}{[Hb]_{tot}}$, the oxygen saturation of haemoglobin

$S' = \dfrac{[HbO_2] + [O_2]_{diss}}{[Hb]_{tot}}$, oxygen saturation of haemoglobin corrected for the physically dissolved oxygen

$\dot{Q}$: cardiac output (1 min^{-1})

q: stroke volume (ml)

f: heart rate (min^{-1})

a and v̄: subscripts denoting arterial and mixed venous blood

A: subscript denoting alveolar

$p_{O_2} = \dot{V}_{O_2}/f$, the oxygen pulse millilitres of oxygen per cardiac beat

P_{CO_2}, P_{O_2}: partial pressures of carbon dioxide and oxygen

$\dot{V}_A$: alveolar ventilation, 1 min^{-1}

$\dot{V}_{CO_2}$: carbon dioxide production, 1 min^{-1} or $\text{ml min}^{-1} \text{ kg}^{-1}$

F_{A,CO_2}: fraction of carbon dioxide in alveolar air

stp: superscript to denote gas at standard conditions, i.e. $0\,°C$, $101\cdot3$ kPa, dryness

H: haemoglobin flow per minute, expressed in litres of oxygen per kilogram body weight per minute.

Since

$$\dot{Q} = f \cdot q, \tag{2.2}$$

from the definition of S and S', eqn (2.1) can be also written

$$\dot{V}_{O_2} = qf[\text{Hb}]_{\text{tot}}(S'_a - S_{\bar{v}}). \tag{2.3}$$

Of these variables $\dot{V}_{O_2}$, f, and $[\text{Hb}]_{\text{tot}}$ are readily determined; S'_a and $S_{\bar{v}}$ may be determined, or alternatively their value may reasonably be assumed. In normal subjects at sea-level S'_a is 0·95–0·98, even during the most strenuous exercise. The saturation of mixed venous blood has been shown to decrease when the oxygen uptake increases, to reach a minimum value of about 0·30 (in male subjects) during the most strenuous exercise, corresponding to a value of $P_{O_2} = 2·53$ kPa, and this value seems to be relatively constant for all individuals. It depends on the minimal P_{O_2} attainable in the tissue and on an appropriate mixture of blood that has perfused the active muscles with that coming from inactive regions. Only in the well-trained individual may this value of the minimal saturation of mixed venous blood possibly drop further to 0·25.

If these assumptions are valid, and assuming further that a maximal heart rate in exercise is 180, then for a maximal workload eqn (2.3) can be simplified to obtain the stroke volume

$$q = 0·00855 \, \dot{V}_{O_2}^{\text{max}} / [\text{Hb}]_{\text{tot}} \tag{2.4}$$

from $\dot{V}_{O_2}^{\text{max}}$ and blood haemoglobin concentration, these data being easily obtained by measurement.

The above assumptions are not of course valid in all cases. For example, at high altitudes, the saturation of the arterial blood is lower than at sea-level, and the correct value must be used in eqn (2.3). On the other hand, when a subject is breathing pure oxygen, the gas physically dissolved in the blood increases from about $3 \, \text{ml} \, \text{l}^{-1}$ when the pressure of oxygen in the alveoli is 100 mm Hg (breathing air at sea-level) to about $18 \, \text{ml} \, \text{l}^{-1}$, and correspondingly more at increased pressure.

In very hot surroundings more blood is driven to the skin to provide greater heat dispersion, and correspondingly less will be available to perfuse the active muscle: $[O_2]_{\bar{v}}$ will then increase and consequently the artero-venous oxygen saturation difference, as well as, from eqn (2.3), the maximal $\dot{V}_{O_2}$, will decrease

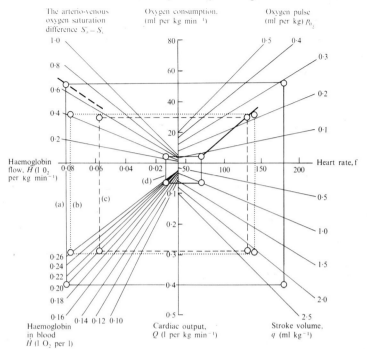

Fig. 2.1. Correlation between oxygen consumption, heart rate, minute-volume of the heart, haemoglobin flow, and other related variables in rest (d); in maximal exercise at sea-level (a); at 5500 m above sea-level (b); and in moderate (60 per cent of maximal) exercise at sea-level (c).

(Lazarovici, Moldovan, Popescu, Nucz, Vracin, and Sac 1970).

The error involved in the assumptions above in calculating q from eqn (2.4) should not be greater than ±5 per cent, which is probably smaller than that affecting the direct measurement. To measure q directly requires an elaborate and time-consuming technique that can be used only in very specialized laboratories. In particular, the method of measuring the cardiac output, which must be accomplished within a circulation time, i.e. within a few seconds, gives results that may differ appreciably from average data obtained over a reasonably long interval of time.

More conveniently than by eqn (2.3), the circulatory variables considered can be described by Fig. 2.1, which is made up of four different coordinate systems placed so that two neighbouring systems have a variable in common. In Fig. 2.1, starting from the upper right and proceeding clockwise the coordinate systems correspond to the following functions:

$$\dot{V}_{O_2} = p_{O_2}f;$$
$$\dot{Q} = qf;$$
$$\dot{H} = [\text{Hb}]_{\text{tot}}\dot{Q};$$
$$\dot{V}_{O_2} = (S'_a - S_{\bar{v}})\dot{H}$$

By plotting on the upper right diagram four experimental points as obtained by recording the heart rate at four oxygen consumption levels (see p. 38) the straight line relating oxygen consumption with heart rate is obtained and this can then be extrapolated to the predetermined value of $f = 180$ to obtain the maximum oxygen consumption. Then by measuring the arterio-venous difference in oxygen saturation, or by assuming that it amounts to 0·65 as described above, the haemoglobin flow $\dot{H}$ expressed in litres of oxygen per kilogram body weight per minute is obtained. If for the oxygen capacity of the blood, we use the value obtained from a haemometric measurement, 0·20 l per l of blood, the volume of blood the heart pumps a minute (minute-volume) and the stroke volume of the blood are also defined, and can be directly read off from the graph.

The *stroke volume* so calculated is the volume at exercise, not at rest. From direct determinations it appears that q increases in exercise up to an oxygen consumption level of about 30 per cent of the maximal aerobic power, to reach a value which does not increase further with increasing work-load even at maximal exercise. The low resting value is possibly due to a residual systolic volume or to an incomplete diastolic filling: the rest volume is not so significant from the functional point of view as the more constant value at exercise.

In old people the maximum heart rate is lower than 180 and the maximum $\dot{V}_{O_2}$ is correspondingly lower. The same is true for people living at high altitude, heart rates as low as 130–140 have been recorded at 5500 m above sea-level (Cerretelli 1961; Pugh, Gill, Lahiri, Milledge, Ward, and West 1964; Cerretelli and Debjiadji 1964).

However, the heart rate for a given submaximal work-load

does not decrease with age, which seems to indicate that in this condition the minute-volume and the stroke volume of the heart are unchanged. The decrease of the maximum heart rate in the old is the reason of the decreased maximum $\dot{V}_{O_2}$: obviously the arteriovenous difference in oxygen saturation is decreased by an amount that is difficult to predict: the value of $0\cdot65$ given above is based on data collected in young, fit individuals in maximal exercise at normal (barometric) pressure.

Were old people able to perform at the same maximum heart rate as the young, the same minute-volume of the heart and the same desaturation of the mixed venous blood would be obtained, with the same actual stroke volume. Therefore to obtain a correct value of q the maximum heart-rate value of 180 together with the value of $0\cdot65$ for the maximum artero-venous saturation difference may also be assumed for old people. When q is obtained, and the maximum heart rate together with the blood capacity for oxygen measured, all the other parameters are easily calculated. For example the condition described as (c) in Fig. 2.1 may well represent the actual effect of age on a subject whose conditions in the youth were described by (a): stroke volume and blood haemoglobin being unchanged, a decrease of the maximum heart rate leads to a decreased $\dot{V}_{O_2}^{max}$ and $\dot{Q}$ together with a decreased arterio-venous difference in blood saturation.

The assumptions made for the oxygen saturation of arterial blood, for the maximal arterio-venous oxygen saturation difference, and for the maximum heart rate may be changed to suit different physiological and pathological conditions, as mentioned earlier. For example in hypoxia, whether due to altitude or to pathological conditions, both S_a and $S_{\bar{v}}$ change substantially, as well as the maximum heart rate. [Hb]$_{tot}$ also undergoes sizable changes, for example after a prolonged sojourn at altitude, as an effect of muscular training or in pathological conditions (anaemia, pletora).

The advantage of the chart of Fig. 2.1 in visualizing the physiological mechanisms involved in particular conditions is evident when changes induced by exercises of different intensity are studied. The lines in Fig. 2.1 have been drawn for the rest conditions and also for maximal exercise at sea-level, for an exercise involving a 60 per cent of the maximum oxygen consumption, and for maximal exercises at an altitude of 5500 m above sea-level which also involves a 60 per cent reduction of the maximum aerobic power.

In my opinion this chart can also be profitably used in clinics, not only to define quantitatively the functional conditions of a subject but also to control objectively the changes induced by a particular therapy or any other treatment.

Once $\dot{V}_{O_2}^{max}$ and q are defined with the help of the chart of Fig. 2.1, other important respiratory characteristics may be assessed; for example the upper and lower diagrams on the left can be replaced by those given in Fig. 2.2. In this the upper diagram relates $\dot{V}_{O_2}$ with the alveolar ventilation.

If the respiratory quotient R.Q. $= [CO_2]/[O_2]$ is known, the values of oxygen consumption on the ordinate may be substituted

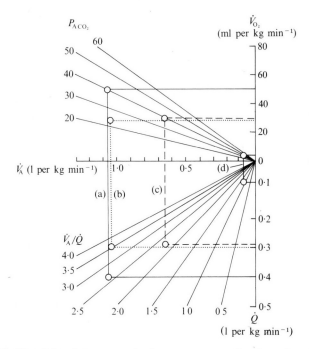

Fig. 2.2. Correlation between maximal oxygen consumption (or carbon dioxide production), alveolar ventilation, minute-volume of the heart, the alveolar partial pressure of carbon dioxide P_{A,CO_2}, and ventilation perfusion quotient under the various experimental conditions as described in Fig. 2.1. Conditions (a), (b), and (c) as in Fig. 2.1.

by those of carbon dioxide production. Let us assume for simplicity that R.Q. is 1, an assumption not too far from reality at the maximum oxygen consumption level; when breathing air, the carbon dioxide contained in inspired air may be neglected, and

$$\dot{V}^{stp}_{CO_2} = \dot{V}^{stp}_A . F_{A,CO_2} \tag{2.5}$$

where F_{A,CO_2} is the fraction of carbon dioxide in alveolar air.

In eqn (2.5) $\dot{V}^{st}_{CO_2}$ and $\dot{V}^{stp}_A$ are volumes in standard conditions (0°C, 101·3 kPa mm Hg, dryness): a correction can be profitably made to reduce $\dot{V}^{stp}_A$ to $\dot{V}^{actual}_A$, i.e. to the actual volume at 37°C, ambient pressure, and saturation with water vapour: a further correction is made to convert F_{A,CO_2} to P_{A,CO_2} the partial pressure of carbon dioxide in alveolar air, resulting in the equation

$$\dot{V}^{stp}_{CO_2} = 0·00116 P_{A,CO_2} . \dot{V}^{actual}_A. \tag{2.6}$$

The upper part of Fig. 2.2 shows $\dot{V}_{CO_2}$ (or $\dot{V}_{O_2}$) as a function of the alveolar ventilation: the lines irradiating from the origin correspond to given P_{A,CO_2} value obtained from eqn (2.6). The lower part of Fig. 2.2 relates the actual alveolar ventilation with the minute-volume of the heart: the isopleths indicate the average ventilation/perfusion ratio $\dot{V}_A/\dot{Q}$ in the lung.

Once $\dot{V}_{O_2}$ and q are known as from Fig. 2.1, it is sufficient to know the value of one of the remaining three variables to obtain the other two. P_{A,CO_2} can easily be measured or, in normal subjects at barometric pressure, it may be assumed constant at about 5·3 kPa even in muscular exercise, as it does not change appreciably with changes of $\dot{V}_{CO_2}$ (Agostoni, Taglietti, and Ferrario Agostoni 1958).

Figure 2.2 clearly shows the effect of exercise on $\dot{V}_A/\dot{Q}$. The increase in $\dot{V}_A$ is much larger than that in $\dot{Q}$, suggesting that in the normal subject the factor limiting maximal exercise is not connected with respiratory mechanics, but lies in the inadequacy of circulatory adaptation. Pulmonary ventilation is also redundant at high altitudes, where the maximum observed values of $\dot{V}_A$ are not appreciably smaller than those at sea-level, in spite of the much lower $\dot{V}^{max}_{O_2}$: this also explains the decreased P_{A,CO_2}.

In conclusion, by measuring
(1) $\dot{V}^{max}_{O_2}$ with the indirect (submaximal exercise) method;
(2) the maximum heart rate at work; and
(3) the blood haemoglobin

we can easily obtain, with the help of Figs 2.1 and 2.2, other significant data such as:

   (a) the arterio-venous oxygen saturation difference;
   (b) the alveolar partial pressure of CO_2;
   (c) the oxygen pulse;
   (d) the stroke volume of the heart;
   (e) the minute-volume of the heart;
   (f) the haemoglobin flow;
   (g) the alveolar ventilation;
   (h) the ventilation/perfusion ratio.

All these data, whose direct determination is very elaborate and restricted to few highly specialized personnel, are of great functional value.

3 Biomechanics of human locomotion

Introduction

It is surprising that human locomotion, which is the most common activity of man and one of the most important and characteristic for his relationship with the external world, was for so long neglected by physiologists. Only in the last decade has satisfactory information and understanding been obtained on its mechanics and on the energy expenditure involved.

For example, it has been known for a long time that walking and running require energy consumption. As the potential energy of a man proceeding on the level at a constant speed does not change, the energy consumed must be dissipated as heat; but how this dissipation takes place, through which intermediate forms of energy, was not known until a few years ago. In 1930 it was generally believed that in running at top speed on the level practically all the energy expenditure was employed to meet the internal viscosity of the muscles, this being the main limit to the speed of progression (see Hill 1927a). It was only after the accurate analysis of the mechanical work involved in running, made by Fenn (1930a) that it was realized that muscle viscosity plays an insignificant role, even when running at top speed.

A sound approach of the study of locomotion first requires the determination of the energy cost of this exercise and secondly a detailed analysis of the mechanical work performed.

The energy cost of walking at a constant speed

An analysis of the energy cost of walking or running can be made in the laboratory by using a treadmill (Fig. 3.1). With this method it is easy to collect the expired air from the subject, and from its analysis the energy expenditure can easily be calculated. Measurements of heart rate, blood collection, etc., can easily be carried out if required.

As the subject has no contact with the outer world except with the belt of the treadmill, which is moving at a constant speed, his

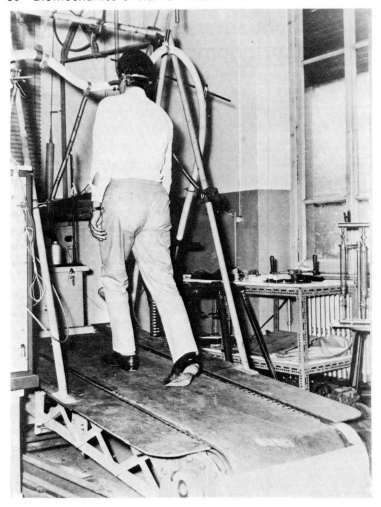

Fig. 3.1. Laboratory treadmill and recording instruments for the study of walking and running.

condition is identical with that of a subject walking or running on the road. The only difference is in the air resistance, which is obviously nil for the subject running on the treadmill; his situation is therefore like that of a man running on the road with a following wind of equal speed.

Subjects at first find some difficulty in walking on a treadmill, and largely because of this some people still think that there is some fundamental difference between walking on the ground and on a treadmill. The difficulties are, however, only psychological and sensory (mainly visual), and are easily overcome with a little training.

The two conditions of walking on a road or on a treadmill are identical because absolute rest cannot be differentiated from motion, at a uniform constant speed: in this situation a condition of absolute rest cannot even be conceived and defined physically. On the other hand everybody knows by experience that on a train or on an aeroplane there is no difference between walking in the same or in the opposite direction as that in which the vehicle is moving. Because the earth rotates around its north–south axis those in temperate latitudes are in fact moving from west to east at a constant speed of about $1500\,\mathrm{km\,h^{-1}}$ (a much higher speed than that reached by the belt of the treadmill!); and walking or running east is certainly no different from progressing west or in any other direction.

The energy cost of walking changes appreciably from subject to subject in relation to body weight. If referred to 1 kg of body weight it is, however, very much the same for all normal subjects as shown in Figs 3.2–3.5, in which the energy expenditure in kilocalories per kilogram and per hour is given as a function of speed for five normal young subjects. Further data for walking

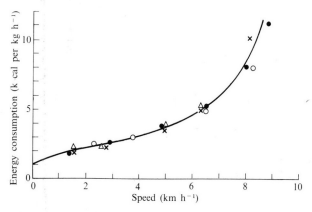

Fig. 3.2. Energy consumption in kilocalories per kilogram of the subject's body weight and per hour (ordinate) walking on the level at different speeds. (From Margaria 1938.)

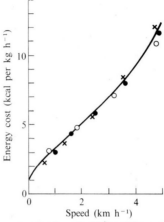

Fig. 3.3. Energy consumption (kcal per kg h^{-1}) walking uphill (+20 per cent) as a function of speed (km h^{-1}).(From Margaria 1938.)

uphill and downhill have been collected for a range of speeds and gradients up to 40 per cent (Margaria 1938).

From these data the energy consumption at rest has been subtracted from the total energy consumption to obtain the *net energy cost* due to the exercise. By further dividing the net energy

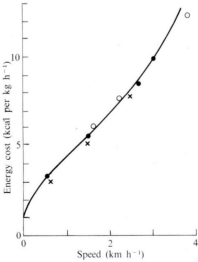

Fig. 3.4. Energy consumption (kcal per kg h^{-1}) walking uphill on an incline of +30 per cent as a function of speed. (From Margaria 1938.)

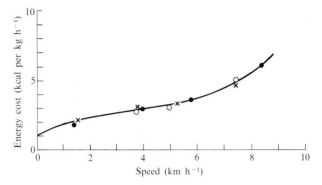

Fig. 3.5. Energy consumption (kcal per kg h^{-1}) walking downhill (-20 per cent) as a function of speed. (From Margaria 1938.)

cost in calories per kilogram per hour by the speed of walking in kilometres per hour *the energy cost per kilogram of body weight and per kilometre* covered has been obtained. These data are summarized in Fig. 3.6.

The energy requirement of walking when the speed and the gradient are known can easily be calculated if the body weight of the subject and the distance covered are known. For example, a man of 70 kg body weight walking 2 km on the level needs $70 \times 2 \times 0 \cdot 5 = 70$ kcal, and the same requirement will be needed for walking back to the point of departure. The energy requirement will therefore total 140 kcal, which can be covered by the administration of about 35 g of sugar or biscuits. To cover the same distance, 2 km, up a 40 per cent gradient will require an energy expenditure of $70 \times 2 \times 3 \cdot 8 = 532$ kcal, and for walking back downhill the energy requirement will be $70 \times 2 \times 0 \cdot 7 = 100$ kcal; the total extra energy expenditure will amount to 632 kcal.

The work-load evidently changes appreciably in walking on an incline, and this should be well considered by those individuals who, because of such functional conditions as anaemia, or heart disease, must keep to a low level of energy expenditure. These data are also valuable for the quantitative treatment of people who take exercise of this kind to reduce their body weight.

Fig. 3.6 indicates that there is an optimum speed at which the energy cost for a given distance covered is minimal: at very low or very high walking speeds the energy requirement increases. This is particularly true for walking uphill up a steep gradient,

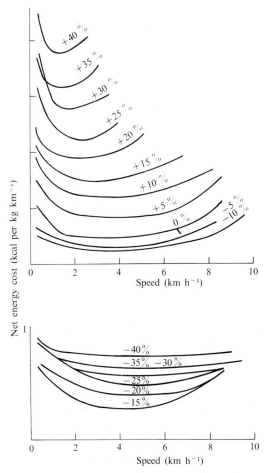

Fig. 3.6. Net energy consumption in walking (kcal per kg km^{-1}) as a function of the speed (km h^{-1}). The incline of the ground is given on each curve. (From Margaria 1938.)

whereas walking on the level and, particularly, downhill the energy requirement is practically independent of speed over a very wide range. For example, walking on the level at speeds from 2 km h^{-1} to 5 km h^{-1} the energy cost remains approximately constant at about 0·5 kcal per kg^{-1} km^{-1}. Walking downhill on −40 per cent gradient the speed range at which the energy cost is the same is even wider, from 2 km h^{-1} to 9 km h^{-1}, the energy requirement being 0·75 kcal per kg^{-1} km^{-1}.

This relative independence of the energy requirement and speed indicates in my opinion that the energy expended in walking is not used meeting frictional resistance such as is met by the foot contacting the ground, or internal resistances such as those due to muscle viscosity: frictional resistances in fact increase appreciably with a moderate increase of speed and the energy expenditure does not increase accordingly.

As the body weight is the product of the mass of the body and the gravitational force, the fact that the energy expenditure per kilogram of body weight is roughly constant indicates that the work performed in walking is largely mass-dependent.

Energy cost of running

The independence of the energy cost for a given distance covered and speed is even more evident in running, at least up to a speed of about 22 km h^{-1} (Margaria 1938; Margaria, Cerretelli, Aghemo, and Sassi 1963a) (Figs 3.7 and 3.8).

Running differs from walking in that the energy requirement

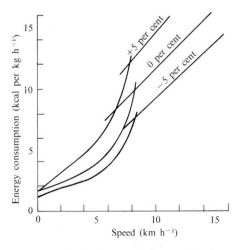

Fig. 3.7. Energy consumption (kcal per kg h^{-1}) in walking (curves at the left) and running (straight lines at the right) on the level, uphill, and downhill at the incline indicated, as a function of speed. (From Margaria 1938.)

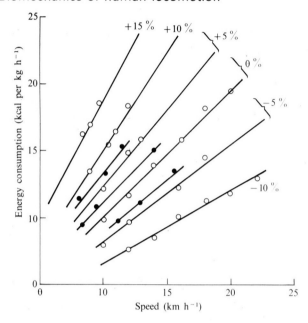

Fig. 3.8. Energy consumption of athletes (full lines) and non-athletes (broken lines) running on the treadmill at the incline indicated. (From Margaria *et al.* 1963.)

per kilogram and per hour in running is a linear function of speed. The slope of the line, which has the significance of the energy cost per kilogram of body weight and per kilometre covered, is constant, i.e. independent of speed. A function analogous to that for walking as represented in Fig. 3.6 would give only a set of lines parallel to the abscissa, one for each gradient.

The mechanical efficiency of walking and running

We consider only the mechanical work represented by the change in the average potential energy of a body progressing at a constant speed, which is solely a function of its vertical displacement. From the energy-consumption data given in Figs 3.6 and 3.8, the mechanical efficiency (= mechanical work/energy consumption) can be calculated for walking at the most economical speed, or when running at any speed (Fig. 3.9).

For *walking on the level* the mechanical efficiency so calculated

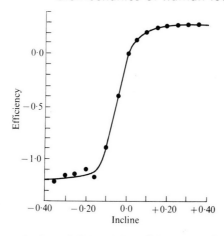

Fig. 3.9. The maximal net 'efficiency' in walking up- or downhill at different inclines of the ground. (From Margaria 1938.)

is obviously nil, because the average potential energy of an individual walking or running on the level at a constant average speed does not change and no mechanical work appears to be performed.

For *walking uphill* the efficiency tends to a value of 0·25, which is reached at a gradient of about 20 per cent. This is the characteristic mechanical efficiency of muscle performing positive work, as is also found in isolated muscle preparations. This finding evidences in my opinion that practically all the work done in walking and running is essentially against gravity.

For *walking downhill* the 'efficiency' so calculated appears to be negative, because the mechanical work performed is negative. The displacement of the body is in the same direction as the gravitational force, opposite to the direction of the force developed by the muscles, and the final energy level of the body is lower than at the start. The energy consumption, on the other hand, is always positive, because when walking downhill muscular activity is still required. The 'efficiency' in this case tends to a value of −1·2, which is reached on a gradient of 10–12 per cent, and this value is also maintained on steeper gradients, of up to −40 per cent (see also Davies and Barnes 1972; Davies, Sargent, and Smith 1974).

Fig. 3.10 shows the energy cost per kilogram and per kilometre

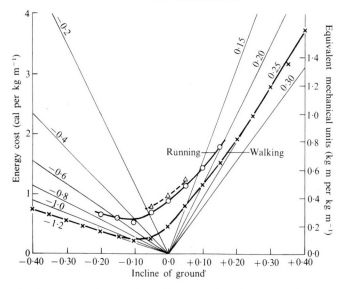

Fig. 3.10. Energy cost (cal per kg, ordinate at left; cal per kg m^{-1}, ordinate at right) for athletes walking at the most economical speed and running as a function of the incline of the ground; (dotted line non athletes). The mechanical efficiency as given by the isopleths irradiating from the origin varies from 0·25 walking uphill, to −1·2 walking downhill. (From Margaria 1963.)

plotted on a coordinate system as a function of the mechanical work due to lifting the body as described above; this is proportional to the gradient when referred to 1 kg of body weight and to 1 km covered. In Fig. 3.10 the isopleths radiating from the origin indicate the efficiencies calculated as described above.

It must be kept in mind that in calculating the mechanical work no consideration has been given to the up-and-down displacement of the body nor to the speed changes that take place at every step: but these tend to be small relative to the total work performed in walking on very steep gradients, both uphill and downhill; they are important only when walking on the level or on very slight gradients.

What appears to me particularly remarkable about Fig. 3.10 is that the energy cost per kilogram and per kilometre turns out to be a linear function of the work as given by the body lift in uphill walking at gradients greater than about 20 per cent, where presumably only positive work is performed: this line coincides with the 0·25 isoefficiency line. For walking downhill a similar linear function is evident for gradients of from −10 per cent to −40 per cent, where presumably only negative work is performed: this line coincides with the isoefficiency line of −1·2.

In other words, in these ranges of gradient the energy consumption is defined by the following simple equations when the work production is known: for walking uphill,

$$E = \frac{E_{mec}}{0·25};$$

for walking downhill,

$$E = \frac{-E_{mec}}{-1·2},$$

where E is the energy consumed and E_{mec} is the positive or negative mechanical work performed (Margaria 1968).

These observations indicate that the energy consumption in these conditions depends only on the work performed against gravity, positive or negative, any other factor being negligible.

When walking on the level at a constant average speed positive and negative work are equal, and the total energy consumed will therefore be

$$E = \frac{+E_{mec}}{0·25} + \frac{-E_{mec}}{-1·2} = \frac{E_{mec}}{0·207}.$$

This equation may be employed to calculate the *mechanical work effectively performed* walking or running on the level when the energy consumption is known.

Positive and negative work

The difference between walking uphill and downhill on steep gradients is substantially due to the fact that uphill walking involves only positive work, and downhill walking only negative work.

Positive work means that accomplished by the muscles against a force, such as gravitation; the active muscles shorten and the potential energy of the system on which the muscles act, i.e. the body mass of the subject, increases. In so-called *negative work*, the displacement of the body is in the opposite direction to the force exerted by the muscles and it takes place in the same direction as the external force acting on the body: the muscle in activity is elongated, and the potential energy of the body, on which the muscle is acting, decreases.

Negative work is a rather awkward term and some people have some difficulty in grasping its meaning. *Potential energy* is defined as the product of the force applied to an object of a given mass and the displacement. When a muscle contracts to lift a weight, this moves in the direction as the force applied by the muscle, and *positive work* is performed. If the weight is too great, and the muscle is unable to lift it, the contraction is *isometric* and the *work is zero.* When the weight of the object is just greater than the muscular force applied to it, work is done on the muscle, which is stretched in the contracted state; the displacement of the object is in the opposite (negative) direction to the muscular force applied: this is considered to be *negative work.* In this case the potential energy of the object decreases; in the case of the lifted weight it increases.

When the muscle contracts to produce *kinetic energy*, as in sprinting or when throwing a weight, the body is accelerated in the same direction as the muscular force applied, and *positive work* is performed. If the muscles in a contracted state are stretched by a moving object, this decelerates; the muscular force acts in an opposite direction to the displacement of the object and the potential energy of this decreases: *negative work* is performed.

In all cases of negative work performed by muscular activity, energy from the outside is absorbed by the muscle and transformed into heat.

The force–velocity diagram of the active muscle

The distinction between positive and negative work is very important in muscle physiology because the force that the muscle can develop during contraction is very different from when it is stretched and then shortens.

The relation between force and speed of contraction is given schematically in Fig. 3.11. A negative velocity of contracting is obviously a velocity of stretching. The velocity of contraction has been studied particularly by Hill (1938). The curve is defined by a somewhat empirical formula which will not be discussed here,

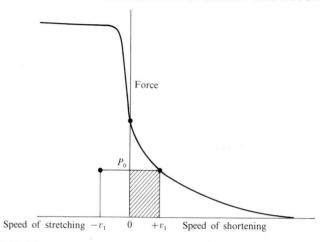

Speed of stretching $-v_1$ 0 $+v_1$ Speed of shortening

Fig. 3.11. Maximal force exerted by a muscle as a function of the speed of shortening (positive values) or of stretching (negative values). The point on the vertical $v = 0$ line indicates the force developed in isometric contraction.

When the load on the muscle is P_0 the maximal speed of shortening is v_1: when the same load is applied on the muscle and its activity graduated in such an amount that stretching occurs, only a fraction of the maximal tension is developed, indicating that only a corresponding fraction of all the contractile elements of the muscle are active.

mainly because it is valid only for the contraction phase and not for stretching.

What appears peculiar in the curve of Fig. 3.11 is the much greater force that an active muscle can develop when stretched and then allowed to shorten than when it is contracting.

Fig. 3.11 can be used to demonstrate important characteristic differences between positive and negative work performances in exercises such as stair-climbing, which involves only positive work, or going downstairs, which involves only negative work. Assuming that in this case the rate of contraction of the muscle is proportional to the speed of progression, then the maximum speed that can be attained in climbing will be $+v_1$ and the mechanical power produced will be given by the dashed area P_0 v_1, where P_0 is the body weight. When walking downstairs at the same speed, $-v_1$, only a fraction of the maximum force that the muscle can develop will be necessary, and correspondingly fewer fibres will be involved; this obviously implies a correspondingly smaller expenditure of energy.

Though the mechanical power involved is the same in positive as in negative work (see Fig. 3.11), the energy expenditure, which presumably depends on the number of the muscle fibres involved, will be less in negative work and its efficiency therefore higher, as shown in Figs 3.9 and 3.10.

The reduction in the force developed by the musle with increasing rate of contraction in positive-work performance was thought to be due to internal muscular viscosity. This theory was, however, soon abandoned. In, particular it was pointed out by Fenn (1930a) that in very rapid muscular contractions, such as take place in fast running, the external work performed is very high, and is of the same order of magnitude as in such activities as uphill walking, which involve slow contractions. The rate of contraction of a muscle when performing positive work was therefore thought to be linked probably to the speed of the chemical reactions involved in activity, and this linked to the force developed according to the force–velocity diagram.

Energy transformations in positive- and negative-work performance

Performing positive work the chemical energy of the muscle is turned into mechanical work, and heat. The mechanical work may in its turn result in an increase in the mechanical energy whether (1) potential, (2) kinetic, or (3) elastic. It may also be employed to overcome internal friction such as (4) muscle viscosity, or friction involved in the deformation of the body, or (5) external friction such as met to overcome the air resistance. In the last two cases the mechanical work is also turned into heat.

The negative work, which may be better visualized as work done on the contracted muscle, is turned (1) into heat, or (2) into elastic energy, which may be eventually used in performing positive work in complex activities, or eventually (3) into chemical energy in the muscle itself were it possible to reverse the chemical exergonic reactions that take place normally in muscle performing positive work (see Maréchal 1964).

The measurement of mechanical work

As mentioned above, when only the potential energy changes of the body are calculated as mechanical work, the mechanical efficiency of locomotion is nil when either walking or running on the level at a constant average speed. In this type of activity—the step cycle, for example—equal amounts of positive and negative work are in fact performed. As a result the net mechanical work accomplished is nil.

Also nil is the work so calculated for a subject stepping on and off a bench or for an individual climbing a set of stairs or a mountain and returning to the starting-point, when only the difference in potential energy of the individual between the end and the beginning of the activity is measured. At the end of the activity the potential energy of the subject is in fact the same as at the starting-point.

For this reason if exact measurements are required of the mechanical work done in activity in which both positive and negative work is performed they must be made at time-intervals that are as small as possible. It will then be apparent that when stepping on a bench, for example, only positive work is performed and when stepping off only negative work is performed. Using still shorter time-intervals, it is easy to show that during walking or running on the level positive work is performed in the first part of the step and is annulled by the negative work performed in the second part of the step. The mechanical work performed at each instant can then be measured exactly, leading finally to a measurement of the total work.

Three methods are available. The oldest method is by stroboscope or cinephotography (see Fig. 3.12). By this method records of the position of the body (trunk and limbs) can be made at very short intervals of time.

Another method is to use an accelerometer fixed to the trunk of the subject. The accelerometer must be sensitive in three directions so that the resultant of the acceleration forces can be obtained, for extent and direction. The force F is easily calculated from the elementary formula

$$F = Ma,$$

where the mass M of the subject is known and the acceleration a measured.

With this instrument reliable results have been obtained for walking. The method is not, however, applicable to running, chiefly because the accelerometer does not remain upright. Because of the oscillations of the trunk of the subject, the axis of

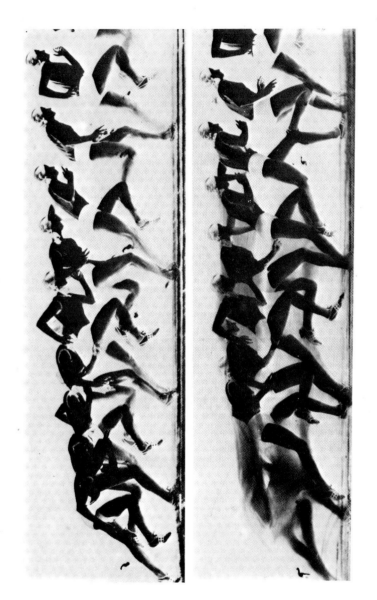

Fig. 3.12. Stroboscopic image of a running man.

reference of the instrument changes continuously, thus making any recording unreliable.

Both these methods measure the displacement or the acceleration of the body or of a given part of it, but not of its centre of gravity, which is the only point representative of the position of the body mass in space. The best method, which gives the resultant of the forces acting on the body directly, is that introduced by Fenn in 1932 with brilliant results. This consists in stepping on a platform that is sensitive to the vertical horizontal, and lateral accelerations, which are recorded graphically. Once the curves of the acceleration as a function of time have been recorded, it is possible by successive integration to obtain the speed changes of the centre of gravity of the body, and finally its displacements.

From the vertical component of the displacement S_V it is easy to calculate the changes in the *potential energy* w_V acquired if the body weight P_0 is known, as

$$W_V = P_0 S_V.$$

From the speed, the *kinetic energy* can be calculated from the well-known equation

$$W_F = \tfrac{1}{2} M v^2.$$

External and internal work

All the work that leads to a displacement of the centre of gravity of the body can be measured with the platform: this is called *external work*. *Internal work* is all the work performed by the muscles that does not displace the centre of gravity of the body.

Internal work may be performed (1) in isometric contractions of the muscles, (2) in meeting friction in the muscles or joints, and (3) in making symmetrical movements of the limbs that do not displace the centre of gravity of the body. Only this last type of internal work may be measured, using the method devised by Fisher in 1911. The displacement and the acceleration of the limbs of a known mass relative to the centre of gravity of the body is measured by means of a stroboscope or cine camera.

As mentioned above, external positive work can easily be measured from the displacement of the centre of gravity of the body in a direction opposite to the force to which it is subjected. The force can be the *gravitational force* (vertical displacements of the centre of gravity of the body) due to the body mass or the inertial forces. Only inertial forces that operate in the direction of movement are important, for the vertical and lateral accelerations are negligible.

Other forces that counteract the movement may be important, for example air resistance or friction with the ground. Normally, however, only the air resistance is likely to be appreciable. In still air the air resistance is appreciable only when running at high speed (see Fig. 3.26).

Potential and kinetic energy changes in walking

The work involved in lifting the body may be defined as *potential* (or antigravitational) *energy* W_V, while that due to acceleration of the centre of gravity of the body in frontal direction is called *kinetic energy* W_F. The *total external work* W_{ext} may be considered to be the sum of those two components.

The ergometers generally used in physiology, such as the treadmill or the cycle-ergometer, register only the work done against an external force contrasting the movement. The platform sensitive to the force exerted by the foot on the ground can measure not only the potential—energy changes, but also the kinetic—energy changes, and therefore all the external work performed. The platform may therefore be considered the most rational ergometer, valid for any type of exercise.

In Fig. 3.13 the results obtained by this method for walking are recorded. The curves (from top to bottom) show the vertical displacement S_V of the centre of gravity of the body, the changes in the potential energy W_V and kinetic energy W_F, and the sum of the potential and kinetic energy changes, W_{ext}.

The curves S_V and W_V are obviously parallel, for they represent the vertical displacement and the potential work, which are directly related by a proportionality factor, which is the body weight of the subject. The curve W_F has been calculated from the body mass and the accelerations in the direction of movement. The vertical and lateral speed changes have been ignored because they are negligible.

It is evident from the curves in Fig. 3.13 that the total external energy change of the body W_{ext} in walking is relatively small, much less than each of its components W_V and W_F. This is due to

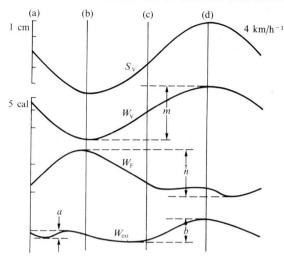

Fig. 3.13. Potential (W_V) and kinetic (W_F) energy changes during a step, walking at a speed of $4 \cdot 0$ km h^{-1}. W_V has been calculated from the vertical displacements of the centre of gravity of the body S_V; W_F from the speed changes in the direction of progression. W_{ext} is the sum of the two curves W_V and W_F; m is the antigravitational work, n the work due to frontal speed changes; $a + b$ is the total external work. (From Cavagna *et al.* 1963.)

the fact that the curves of the potential and kinetic energy changes are substantially opposite in phase.

This suggests that the increase of kinetic energy in a certain phase of the step takes place at the expense of the potential energy, which at the same time decreases, and vice versa. The lifting of the body in the first phase of the step when walking slowly does not contribute directly to the forward displacement of the body, but it may be utilized to this end in the second part of the step during the falling forward of the body. The increased kinetic energy that the body thus acquires may in its turn be utilized in the first phase of the next step to lift the body, thus saving some of the work that the limb muscles would have to accomplish to this end.

A mechanical model of walking

If we imagine an egg rolling end over end on a smooth horizontal surface (see Fig. 3.14), the displacement of its centre of gravity in a vertical plane will be similar to that of the curve S_V in Fig. 3.13.

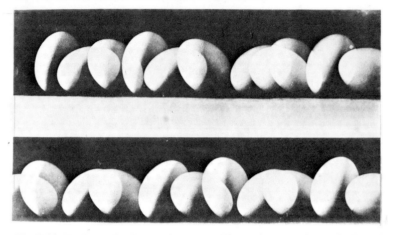

Fig. 3.14. Stroboscopic picture of an egg rolling end over end on a horizontal surface (see text).

The speed in the direction of the progression will also oscillate from a minimum value when the centre of gravity of the egg is at its highest point to a maximum value when it is at its lowest. The changes of the kinetic and potental energy of the rolling egg will be represented by curves similar to the curves W_F and W_V in Fig. 3.13. These curves would be regular sine curves in exactly opposite phase. Their sum, W_{ext}, would therefore be represented by a horizontal line parallel to the abscissa in the ideal case when energy is not lost by friction and the egg receives no energy from outside.

If the energy is consumed in friction of some sort however, the kinetic energy of the egg when its centre of gravity is at its lowest will not be enough to raise the centre of gravity to its highest point. Energy must then be furnished by a force that we may imagine to be directed vertically. This energy would be represented by an upward displacement of the curve W_{ext}, such as *a* and *b* in Fig. 3.13.

The *rolling egg* is a good model of human walking, though perhaps a little too simple. In walking at low speed the push of the foot on the ground due to muscular activity is substantially directed vertically; the body is lifted and the potential energy increased. This potential energy is transformed into kinetic energy in the second phase of the step, when the body is leaning forward. The falling forward of the body, which is assisted by the skeletal levers and by muscle tone, is arrested when the other foot is brought forward and strikes the ground. The centre of gravity of the body is then lifted again, mostly at the expense of the kinetic energy acquired during the falling phase of the step.

High-speed walking

A deviation from this model is observed in high-speed walking. The push of the foot on the ground is then directed not only upward, but also forward; it acquires a frontal component that is greater the higher the speed of progression (Fig. 3.15).

Obviously the increase of the potential energy at each step is limited by the anatomical dimensions and by the architecture of the body, particularly that of the foot. It cannot therefore be further increased when the speed of walking is increased above certain values, and an increase of kinetic energy is required. At speeds higher than about 5 km h^{-1} the only way to increase the speed of progression is to increase the forward component of the push of the foot on the ground, which is negligible when walking at low speed.

In Fig. 3.16 the potential energy, kinetic energy, and total external work performed in walking are given as a function of the speed of progression. Up to a speed of about 6 km h^{-1}, the potential energy changes are greater than the kinetic ones, and these may therefore take place at the expense of the first. At speeds above above about 7 km h^{-1} the potential energy changes at each step do not increase further with increasing speed of progression: on the contrary, they decrease progressively while the kinetic energy increases with increasing increment.

The total energy changes that take place at each step in walking at low speed occur in two distinct phases. These are shown in Fig. 3.13 by a, in which a forward push is presumably given to the body, particularly by the activity of the gastrocnemius and soleus muscles, and b, which is due to the activity of the glutei that extend the thigh relative to the trunk, thus raising the centre of gravity of the body.

In high-speed walking these two phases tend to sum up in one phase only, and the curve of the total energy changes tends to approach more and more the curve of the kinetic energy changes.

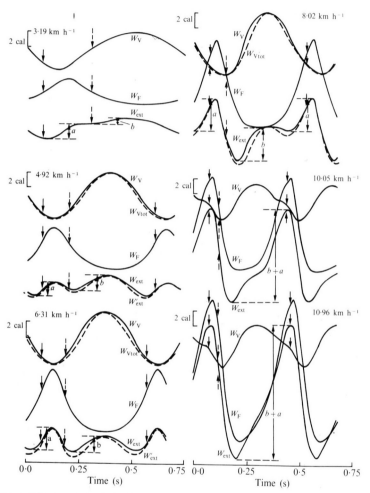

Fig. 3.15. Potential (W_V), kinetic (W_F) and total (W_{ext}) energy changes in cal (2 cal per mark) at different speeds of walking as indicated. W_{vtot} (broken line) is the total energy change due to the vertical displacement, including beside W_V the kinetic energy changes involved in the upward movement. (From Cavagna and Margaria 1966.)

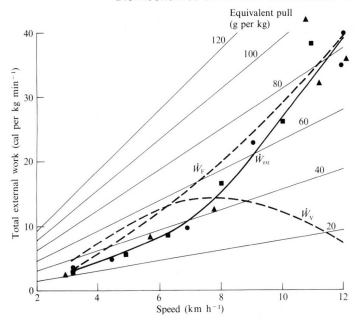

Fig. 3.16. Total external work W_{ext} in walking, in calories per kg of body weight per minute, as a function of the average speed of progression (full line). The broken lines are the single components W_F (work necessary to sustain the velocity changes) and $\dot{W}_V$ (work performed against gravity), of the resultant $\dot{W}_{ext}$. Different symbols refer to three different subjects. (From Cavagna and Margaria 1966.) The lines radiating from the origin have been added: the numbers on them indicate the mechanical work in gram metres per m covered and per kilogram of body weight, or the equivalent pull in grams per kilogram . (From Margaria 1968.)

The mechanics of running

The mechanics of running is substantially different from that of walking at moderate speed. Running is characterized by a push of the foot on the ground necessarily directed both upward and forward, not only upward, as in low-speed walking. The potential energy of the body W_V increases together with the kinetic energy W_F.

As can be seen from Fig. 3.17, the curves W_F and W_V are substantially in phase, and the amplitude of the curve W_{ext} representing the oscillations of the total external energy of the body is the sum of the changes of its two components: i.e., it is much higher than the amplitude of its two single components, in

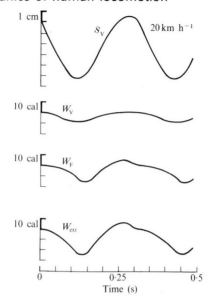

Fig. 3.17. Vertical displacement of the centre of gravity S_V, and changes in potential energy W_V, kinetic energy W_F and total energy W_{ext} during a single step when running at 20 km h^{-1}. (From Cavagna *et al.* 1964.)

contrast to the situation during walking. Therefore, it seems that in running it is not possible to change kinetic into potential energy or vice versa, as in walking.

This also explains the much higher energy expenditure involved in running, as is evident from Figs 3.6, 3.8, 3.9, and 3.10. Whereas the energy cost of walking on the level at the most economical speed is about 0·5 cal per kg m^{-1}, that for running is twice as much, about 1 cal per kg m^{-1}.

The potential energy acquired at each step in walking may be utilized for forward progress, but in running only the horizontal component of the push of the foot on the ground is effective for progress. The potential energy acquired in running is therefore effectively wasted, but it may be regarded as necessary to the mechanics of running.

Another fundamental characteristic of running is that the *vertical component of the push* of the foot on the ground has a value equal to the body weight (Fig. 3.18), and it is a constant independent of speed. Only the horizontal component of the push

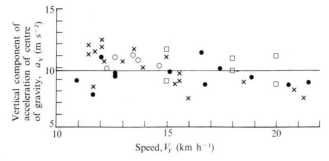

Fig. 3.18. Vertical component of the acceleration of the centre of gravity of the body at each step (ordinate) when running at different speed. The horizontal line indicates the value of the acceleration of gravity (9.81 m sec^{-2}). Different symbols correspond to different subjects. (From Cavagna *et al.* 1964.)

increases with increasing speed. In other words, the direction of the force exerted by the foot on the ground is more inclined forward at high speed (Fig. 3.19) and the angle that it makes with the horizontal decreases progressively to reach a minimum value of about 45° in top sprinting (such as is observed at the start of a 100-m race). A smaller angle, i.e. a more forward push, is incompatible with the mechanics of running because the foot would slip on the ground; this is why sprinters use nailed shoes.

Obviously on icy or on sandy soils where the coefficient of friction is less, the minimum angle of the push may be much higher than 45°, and may approach 90°.

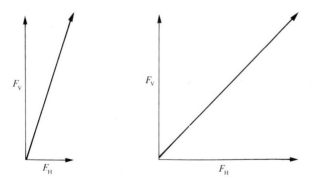

Fig. 3.19. Magnitude and direction of the push of the foot on the ground running at low (left) and high (right) speed. The vertical component F_V has the same value, equal to g: only the horizontal component F_H increases with increasing speed.

As shown in Fig. 3.18, in running the centre of gravity of the body is never lifted above the position it has when the subject is standing in the erect position: in *jumping*, on the contrary, the vertical acceleration conferred to the body by the limb muscles is greater than the gravitational acceleration and the centre of gravity of the body is correspondingly raised. Jumping is therefore fundamentally different from running. The vertical component of the push given at every step by the runner is equal to the gravitational acceleration and such that the body just floats for an instant in the air, while the legs are flexed and the feet are off the ground. In this instant the body is still subjected to the gravitational force and the centre of gravity is displaced forward and downward. When the forward foot strikes the ground, because of the skeletal levers the displacement of the centre of gravity of the body changes direction, bending upward.

When the foot strikes the ground the body is subjected to a deceleration, which is due to the force exerted by the ground on the subject. Its direction is upward and backward from the point of contact of the foot on the ground to the centre of gravity of the body: the backward component is responsible for the deceleration. The deceleration due to this factor and the deceleration due to the air resistance met during the floating phase are the two components of the total deceleration encountered at each step.

As mentioned above, the vertical component of the push of the foot on the ground in running is not utilized for forward progress: it is, so to speak, a technical necessity because it is not possible to give a purely horizontal push. There must be a vertical component, which will be larger in relation to the horizontal component the more slippery the ground.

The phases of the potential and kinetic energy changes in walking and running

The phase relationship of the potential and kinetic energy oscillations in walking and running may be described by plotting on a coordinate system for a subject walking or running on a treadmill at a constant average speed the vertical and the horizontal displacements of the centre of gravity of the body relative to the position it would have at constant speed.

These functions are represented in Fig. 3.20. If the vertical and horizontal displacements of the centre of gravity of the body were

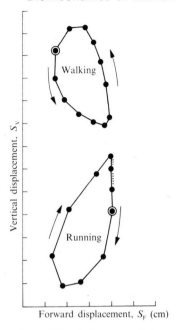

Fig. 3.20. Vertical S_V and frontal S_F displacement of the centre of gravity of the body in a subject walking or running on a treadmill. All the points are at $1/30$ s interval. The larger point on each contour marks the moment at which heel touches the ground. In two dotted intervals of the contour for running the subject has no contact with the ground. (From Cavagna *et al.* 1964.)

in perfect phase this function would be represented by a straight line directed upward and to the right (top of Fig. 3.21). If the two variables were in exactly opposite phase the function would also be represented by a straight line, but in this case directed downward and to the right. If the difference of phase were 90° or 270°, the function would be represented by a circle. In fact for both walking and running we do have neither a straight line nor a circle, but something in between, namely a cycloid (Fig. 3.20).

For running, the greater axis of the cycloid is directed upward and to the right, indicating that the two variables tend to be in phase. In general a vertical displacement of the centre of gravity corresponds to a displacement forward and vice versa. Only in one segment (each segment corresponds to $\frac{1}{30}$ s) is there a backward displacement of the centre of gravity corresponding to a

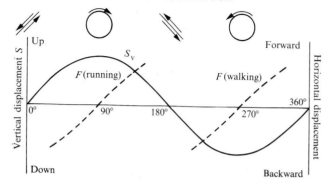

Fig. 3.21. Vertical displacement of a body subjected to a vertical pendular movement (ordinate at left) against time. If the body is subjected simultaneously to another indentical pendular movement directed horizontally (ordinate at right) the path drawn at the top of the Figure is described by the body on a sagittal plane, depending on the phase difference between the two movements. Values on the abscissa indicate the difference of phase. Broken lines indicate the frontal pendular component that together with the vertical component S_V would result in a circular figure. Walking is more near the condition described by the left-hand line, running by the right-hand line. (From Cavagna *et al.* 1964.)

vertical displacement. Only in this short interval of time, therefore, is a change of potential into kinetic energy or vice versa possible. It is possible to calculate from the graph that the phase difference between the vertical and horizontal displacement is about 20°.

The cycloid relating to walking has its major axis directed downward and to the right, indicating that a lowering of the centre of gravity takes place at essentially the same time as a forward displacement, i.e. that the two variables are in opposite phase. The phase difference is about 200° in this case, only 20° from opposing phase. As in running, only one segment of the cycloid is directed upward and to the right, and only in this short interval of time is there no possibility of transformation of kinetic into potential energy or vice versa.

A mechanical model of running

The egg rolling end over end on the level is evidently not an acceptable mechanical model for running, which is more like the progress of an elastic bouncing ball (Fig. 3.22). In this case the push is given by the elastic recoil of the ball, which has been

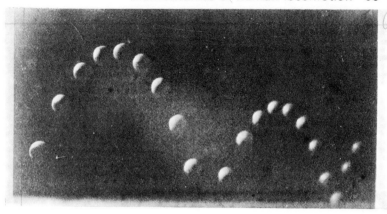

Fig. 3.22. Stroboscopic images of a bouncing ball as a model of running. The upper and forward push to the ball is given by the elastic energy stored in the ball when this strikes the ground. Elastic energy is similarly stored in the muscles and tendons of the lower limbs at the end of each step in running and can be utilized as kinetic and potential energy in the next step.

deformed by its impact with the ground. This force, as in running, is directed upward and forward.

This model is fairly realistic, in that in running elastic energy is stored in the muscles and tendons when the foot strikes the ground: this elastic energy is immediately given back as potential and kinetic energy, at the beginning of the next step, and is added to the energy due to the activity of the contractile components of the muscle. At the moment of the impact of the foot on the soil the extensors muscles of the lower limbs are in fact actively contracted to prevent bending of the joints of the limbs under the weight of the upper part of the body and the inertial forces. In this condition the muscles accumulate elastic energy.

The ability of muscle to accumulate elastic energy and to utilize it in the performance of positive work as described above has always been denied by physiologists in the past. Fenn (1930b, 1957) and Elftman (1944–66) in particular considered as negligible the utilization of the elastic energy by the muscle. The mechanical efficiency in high-speed running was found by Fenn to be very high, approaching 25 per cent. This is equal to the overall maximum efficiency of muscular contraction due to the activity of the contractile elements of the muscle. There was therefore thought to be no room for any contribution from elastic energy, which by saving a corresponding amount of chemical energy would have resulted in an increase of the mechanical efficiency. Furthermore, they argued that as only muscle in a state of contraction can accumulate elastic energy and as the maintenance of a condition of activity requires energy expenditure, an appreciably higher efficiency could not have been reached. In other words, the cost of maintaining the contraction could not have been appreciably less than the gain acquired by utilizing the elastic energy. These arguments are disproved by the finding that efficiency in running can be much higher than 25 per cent, as described in detail in the following chapter.

The mechanical efficiency of running

The importance of the elastic energy that can be stored in the muscle in activity, and its amount in activities in which rapid contractions and relaxations are required, was established with certainty only by exact measurements of the mechanical work involved in running, using the method previously described (p. 83).

From data on the external work per kilogram and per minute as a function of the speed both when walking and running (Figs 3.16, 3.17, and 3.23) the external work per kilometre and per kilogram of body weight has been calculated (Fig. 3.24). The energy cost of walking and running being known, the mechanical efficiency can then be calculated.

When walking and running on the level at a constant speed, positive and negative work are equal. The efficiency for the positive work is 0.25 and that for negative work is -1.2. The overall efficiency is 0.207 (see p. 77). In Fig. 3.24 the energy cost of the exercise is given with a scale five times larger (ordinate at right) than for the data of external work (kcal per kg km^{-1}) (ordinate at left). If the mechanical efficiency were 0.2, the lines indicating the energy expenditure (ordinate at right) should pass through the experimental points for the mechanical work data.

For walking, the data for external work are in fact slightly below the energy expenditure curve, which indicates that the mechanical efficiency in this case is very little lower than the assumed value of 0.2. For running, on the contrary, the data for mechanical work are appreciably above the line for energy consumption,

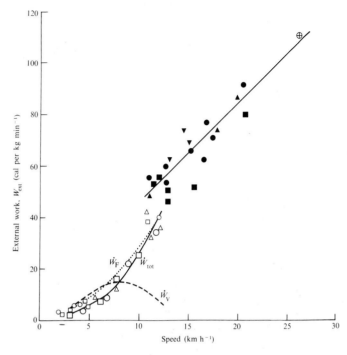

Fig. 3.23. External work per kilogram of body weight and per minute in walking (lower curves at left) and running (upper straight line) on the level at a constant average speed of progression (full lines). Broken lines indicate the components $\dot{W}_V$ and $\dot{W}_F$ of $\dot{W}_{ext}$ in walking. (From Cavagna 1969.)

showing that the average efficiency in this exercise is appreciably greater than 0·20: about 0·25.

The internal work must also be taken into consideration in running. By adding the internal work to the external work as measured from moving-picture analysis, in running, the total work performed is obtained, and this is indicated by the broken line on the top of Fig. 3.24 (W_{tot}) (Cavagna et al. 1964).

This value of total mechanical work represents a very high mechanical efficiency of about 0·4 or more. This is much higher than the maximum value for the efficiency of muscular contraction even in purely positive work as walking uphill (0·25), where the necessarily slow movements and the optimum frequency of contractions greatly reduce the possibility of loss of energy

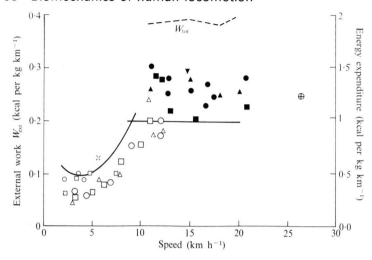

Fig. 3.24. Experimental data of external mechanical work (kcal per kg km^{-1}) in walking and running for different subjects (left ordinate) as a function of speed, as from the data of Fig. 3.23. The broken line on top of figure gives the data of total mechanical work W_{tot} (external and internal) for the same subjects. The full lines give the energy expenditure (kcal per kg km^{-1}) in walking and running (ordinate at right). (From Cavagna 1969.)

through muscle viscosity or accessory muscular contraction not directly utilized.

Such a high value of mechanical efficiency evidently must involve an error in the calculation of the efficiency as conventionally defined by

$$E = \frac{\text{mechanical work}}{\text{energy consumption}}.$$

As the measurement of the energy consumption in running is easy and reliable, the error could originate in an overestimate of the positive mechanical work performed by the muscles. The data obtained in our experiments seemed, however, very accurate and reproducible and the possibility of a technical error of such magnitude was out of the question. Furthermore, similar data had been obtained by Fenn many years previously (1930a) in a subject running at 27 km h^{-1}. The only source of error in calculating the efficiency could be if the positive mechanical work were performed at the expense of some other source in addition to the chemical energy as measured from the energy consumption. Therefore the hypothesis has been put forward that elastic energy could be stored in the muscle in the negative work phase that immediately precedes the performance of positive work. This could be a consequence of the stretching of the elastic structures (muscles and tendons) under the weight of the body and inertial forces. Similarly, in the bouncing ball, as indicated in Fig. 3.22, the changes in potential and kinetic energy are not due to any chemical energy but only to the elastic energy that is acquired by the deformation of the ball when it strikes the ground.

Fenn was surprised by the very high value of the mechanical efficiency, about 0.25, that he found in running. This value is, however, appreciably less than that found in the experiments described above. The discrepancy is presumably due to the fact that Fenn did not measure directly the energy expenditure of the subject. He made use of the data obtained by Sargent in 1926 in short sprints at maximum speed, which entailed an energy expenditure much higher than is reached when running at a steady speed. Sargent measured the oxygen consumption during the exercise and for a long period during recovery and subtracted from this the pre-exercise rest value. This method has been criticized by Margaria et al. (1934) and by Lloyd (1966). It is in fact liable to give an overestimate because it does not take account of an appreciable increase in the rest oxygen consumption value as an effect of heavy muscular exercise. This increased oxygen consumption has no direct connection with the mechanism of energy exchanges such as those involved in the contraction and payment of the oxygen debt (see p. 30). Sargent's data have furthermore not been confirmed by other authors, who have recorded much lower values of oxygen consumption.

The total positive external work performed in walking and running is thus not given only by the sum of the potential and kinetic energy changes as indicated in Figs. 3.15 and 3.16. To these two components a third should be added: the curve of the elastic energy changes W_{el}. This, however, cannot be measured. The curve would show a maximum when W_V and W_F are at a minimum, namely when the extensor muscles of the lower limbs are stretched in a state of contraction, to damp the impact of the body on the ground; and it would show a minimum when the foot leaves the ground, when W_V and W_{kin} are at a maximum, and the pull by the muscles in contraction does not meet any further resistance due to the body weight and to the inertial forces. Only if it were possible to obtain a W_{tot} curve as the sum of these three curves would the mechanical work done by the muscles be representative of the chemical changes that have taken place as an effect of the contraction.

It may seem surprising that the importance of the elastic energy in muscular exercise was not discovered earlier by physiologists. The magnitude of the elastic energy utilized in running is in fact very appreciable, and is nearly equal to the energy given by the contracting elements of the shortening muscles. And the term 'elastic' recurs very frequently in the terminology of laymen, such as athletes, trainers, or the public in general to describe the movement and the performance of athletes.

External and internal resistances in walking and running

We observed above that: (a) the energy cost per kilogram of body weight and per metre covered in walking is constant for a wide range of speeds, particularly when walking on the level or downhill, and it is wholly independent of speed in running: and (b) the efficiency of walking at the most economical speed has about the value that would be calculated on the assumption that in positive work the efficiency is 0.25 (as found on the isolated muscle) and that in negative work is -1.2. In my opinion these observations indicate that the energy spent walking on the level is substantially due to the production of mechanical work, positive or negative, implied in lifting and lowering the body and in the acceleration and deceleration that take place at each step. Any other factor, except perhaps air resistance, appears to be inappreciable.

We can draw the conclusion that muscular viscosity, which in the 1920s was given a very high importance as a limiting factor in running, has on the contrary no appreciable importance. If muscular viscosity were an important factor, as the friction increased at high speed, the energy cost would also be greatly influenced as the contraction of the muscles would be faster. In reality, as stated above, speed of running has no appreciable effect on the energy cost for running a given distance.

Though this appears to be the most simple and logical explanation for the independence of the energy cost per kilometre and kilogram of body weight and the speed in running, the possibility that this could be the resultant of the compensation of an actual negative effect due to muscular viscosity, increasing with speed, and a positive effect due to a greater utilization of muscular elasticity cannot be excluded.

The resistance to progression can therefore be considered as substantially due to the negative work that is performed at each step in walking and running: to maintain a constant speed of progression this must be compensated by an equal amount of positive work. It has been found that in walking the deceleration taking place at each step increases linearly with the speed of progression: this explains the increased cost of fast walking (Cavagna and Margaria 1966).

Of the external resistances met in walking and running, only those due to the friction of the foot on the ground and to air resistance are appreciable.

External friction resistances

The friction due to the first contact of the foot on the ground is very small or non-existent, because in the phase immediately preceding the contact of the foot on the ground, the foot is accelerated backwards, and its speed relative to the ground is reduced to zero or even a slightly negative value: in the latter case a very small forward acceleration is given to the body (see Fig. 3.25). If the wheels of a landing aircraft were put in motion to a speed of rotation corresponding to the speed at landing before they touched the ground, they would exert no breaking action touching the ground and no tearing of the tyres would take place. Similarly, in both walking and running the foot does not strike the ground tangentially but it just lies on it, thus avoiding any frictional resistance.

Air resistance has been measured experimentally by recording the pressure exerted by the air on a model of man in different positions in a wind tunnel (Du Bois-Raymond 1925; Hill 1927b). These authors found that the pressure F on the model increased with the square of the speed of the wind v, namely

$$F = kv^2.$$

The power $\dot{W}$ necessary to overcome this force per second is

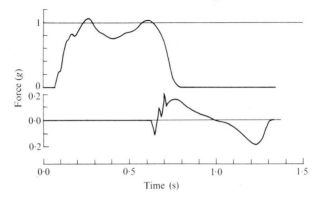

Fig. 3.25. Vertical (upper) and forward (lower) directed forces expressed in multiples of gravitational force g as a function of the time, obtained by stepping with a single foot on the two platforms, one sensitive to the vertical and one to the forward forces. Walking speed 4·5 km h^{-1}. (From Cavagna and Margaria 1966.) On the tracing for the platform sensitive to forward forces, at the first contact of the foot on the ground a very short forward push is recorded, soon followed by the deceleration and in the second part of the step by a sustained forward push, responsible for the positive work performance.

therefore

$$\dot{W} = F \times v = kv^3;$$

it increases with the third power of the wind velocity.

By expressing the power in kilograms metres per kilogram of body weight per second, and the speed in metres per second it has been found experimentally that $k = 0.00035$.

The curve of Fig. 3.26 plots this function ($\dot{W} = 0.00035v^3$) against speed. These data have also been confirmed by Fenn (1930), who found the work due to the air resistance by measuring the difference between the acceleration and the deceleration taking place at each step: the deceleration due to the impact of the foot on the ground was always less than the acceleration previously conferred to the body, because some kinetic energy was lost due to the air resistance met in the flight phase.

The isopleths in Fig. 3.26 are the iso-resistance lines. It can easily be seen that when running at a speed of 10 m s^{-1} the air resistance is 35 g per kg of body weight. The same effect could be obtained in still air (on the treadmill) by a backward pull of the same magnitude or more simply by inclining the treadmill by 3·5 per cent. In general the data of Fig. 3.26 can be used to assess the

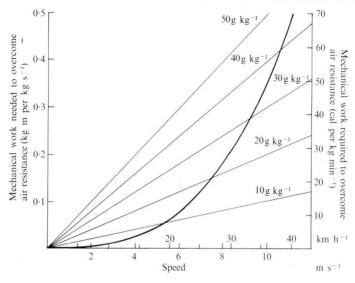

Fig. 3.26. The mechanical work required to overcome air resistance (left ordinate: kg m per kg s^{-1}; right ordinate: cal per kg min^{-1} as a function of the speed of progression. The numbers on the isopleths irradiating from the origin give the equivalent pull in grams per kilogram of body weight. (From Margaria 1968.)

incline of the treadmill needed to reproduce the effect of any value of air resistance, when walking and running at a given speed in still air.

As shown in Fig. 3.26, the air resistance running or walking at speeds of up to 10 km h^{-1} is insignificant.

'Wasted' mechanical work in locomotion

The positive work necessary to compensate for the negative work utilized to maintain a constant speed does not increase the average potential energy of the body; from this point of view it may therefore be considered as 'wasted'. This positive, 'wasted' work in fact constitutes all the work performed when walking or running on the level at a constant speed: on an incline the potential energy increases walking uphill and decreases walking downhill.

For a small uphill incline, there is still some wasted work because the vertical displacement of the body at each step is greater than that necessary to move up the incline. Only when the incline of the ground is greater than 20 per cent is the lift of the body at each step not followed by an appreciable lowering of the centre of gravity of the body in the second phase of the step. Also, the deceleration taking place at each step becomes inappreciable, because uphill walking is usually at a relatively low speed: negative work is therefore no longer performed.

Similarly, walking downhill, at an incline greater than 10 per cent the body is not lifted at each step nor is muscular activity necessary to accelerate the body, this being promoted only by the gravitational force. All the work performed is therefore negative.

In Fig. 3.10 the energy expenditure necessary to meet this 'wasted' work is represented by the distance between the oxygen consumption curve at a given incline value and the iso-efficiency lines indicated 0·25 for uphill walking and −1·2 for downhill walking. The distance between these iso-efficiency lines and the abscissa gives the change, gain or loss, in the potential energy of the body at a given incline. The energy wasted in walking and running, on the level, uphill, and downhill, is given in Fig. 3.27. It appears that, walking on the level, the mechanical work wasted amounts to $0·044 \text{ kg m per m}^{-1}$.

The value for the wasted positive work for walking on the level as calculated from the data of energy consumption and the efficiency ($= 0·207$) is only very slightly greater than the value for

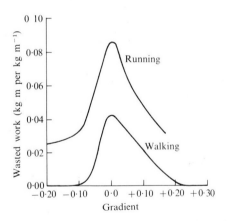

Fig. 3.27. 'Wasted' work (negative work performed when going uphill or positive work when going downhill) walking at the most economic speed or running. Abscissa: incline of the ground: +uphill, −downhill. (From Margaria 1968.)

mechanical work measured directly with the platform: this supports the hypothesis mentioned earlier that the energy consumed in walking on the level at moderate speed is practically all employed in performing positive and negative external work, an inappreciable amount being employed to perform internal work (friction, viscosity, isometric contractions, etc.). However, this internal work increases very appreciably with increasing speed of walking, to reach a value about half the external positive work performed when walking at $8.5 \, km \, h^{-1}$.

Running on the level the wasted work is twice as much as in walking, amounting to twice the total energy consumption per kilogram of body weight per kilometre. This is due to the fact that in walking the potential positive work performed in the first half of the step is utilized for the progression while in running potential energy cannot be transformed into kinetic energy.

Running uphill the wasted work decreases, but it is never reduced to zero as in walking, probably (a) because as running is at high speeds of progression it cannot take place at very large inclines as can walking, as this would require an oxygen consumption greater than the maximum; and possibly also because (b) the internal work in running may be appreciable even at a reduced speed.

Running downhill, the wasted work decreases to less than the half its maximum value at an incline of 10 per cent. At greater incline values data are lacking because of technical difficulties involved when running on a treadmill mainly that the belt of the treadmill changes speed every time the foot strikes the ground (see also the recent paper by Davies *et al.* (1972)).

In conclusion, the 'resistance' met by the subject when walking or running on the level appears to be essentially met by the negative work that is performed at each step which must be compensated by an equal amount of positive work in the first phase of the following step: practically all the energy spent in walking and running on the level is utilized to meet this resistance.

The wheel model of human locomotion

As mentioned earlier, the negative work performed at each step is substantially that caused by the deceleration of the body when the forward foot strikes the ground. At that moment the body will be subjected by a force F directed upwards and backwards from the point of contact of the foot on the ground, towards the centre of gravity of the body. The horizontal component of this force F_H leads to a decrease in the kinetic energy of the body: F_H will decrease the higher the speed of progression and the higher the angle α that the force F makes with the horizontal, to tend to zero when α tends to $90°$ ($\cos 90° = 0$).

Let us imagine a rimless wheel, made only of spokes: the more spokes there are the smoother this wheel will run on a flat surface. If the number of spokes is infinite, i.e. the wheel is a disc, or if the wheel is provided with a rim, it will roll perfectly smoothly on a flat surface.

Let us imagine a wheel made up of only four spokes: when each of these strikes the ground, the wheel will be subjected to a force from the point of contact of the spoke on the ground directed upward and backward (see Fig. 3.28(a)). The backward (horizontal) component F_H will decrease with an increasing number of spokes, because at the moment the spoke strikes the ground the line between the centre of gravity of the wheel and the point of the contact on the ground will be more nearly vertical, and the angle α will increase. In a wheel with an infinite number of spokes or in an ordinary wheel provided with a rim, the centre of gravity of the wheel will be exactly vertically above the point of contact of the spoke on the ground: the horizontal

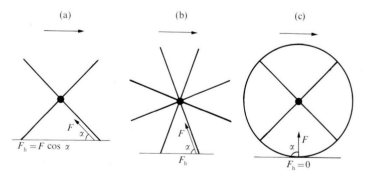

Fig. 3.28. A rimless wheel will be subjected to a backward force defined by $F \cos \alpha$ every time a spoke strikes the ground. This force will decrease by increasing the number of spokes and become nil when this number is infinite, or in a wheel provided with a rim (c).

component F_H ($= F \cos \alpha$) will be zero and the wheel can proceed freely.

This model is illustrated in Fig. 3.28. The negative work is decreasing from (a) to (c). The same effect may be obtained in running, so decreasing the main effective resistance to progression. The positive work performed can then be utilized to increase the kinetic energy of the body in motion rather than being wasted to neutralize negative work. To shift from model (a) to the (b) or (c) of Fig. 3.28 the runner should take shorter and more frequent steps. In practice it is not easy to reach this goal because when running at top speed on the level a frequency of 5 steps per second is reached and this is possibly the highest limit of frequency for this exercise: the speed of shortening of the muscles cannot be increased further at the force values required. An increased speed of contraction would in fact lead necessarily to a decreased force, as described by the well-known force–speed diagram of contraction (Fenn and Marsch 1935; Hill 1938; Wilkie 1950) (see also Fig. 3.11).

A higher step frequency in running, together with a shorter step stride, is however realized spontaneously in the initial acceleration phase of an all-out sprint, as is shown in Fig. 3.29. In fact the maximal step frequency is reached after the first few steps, when the speed of progression is not very high: the steps are necessarily very short, and the foot strikes the ground when the centre of gravity of the body is nearly on the vertical of the point of contact of the foot with the soil as in the case of the conventional full wheel (Fig. 3.28(c)) there is practically no deceleration, and all the mechanical energy liberated by the muscle may be employed to increase the kinetic energy of the subject, to perform positive work.

But when the speed of progression increases a reduction of the step length would involve an intolerable increase of the step frequency, as is shown clearly by Fig. 3.29.

From the considerations above one might expect the energy cost of running for quadrupeds to be greater than that for man: the centre of gravity of the body is in fact displaced backward relative to the front limbs, which strike the ground at the end of the step. The energy cost per kilogram of body weight and per metre covered for dogs progressing at low speed is about twice as high as that for a walking man (Cerretelli *et al.* 1963; Stegemann

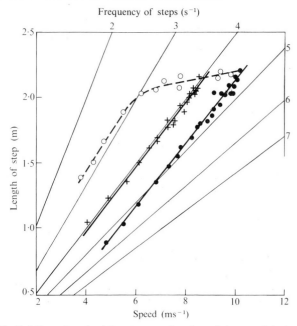

Fig. 3.29. Full lines: length of the step as a function of the speed during a sprint at top speed in two Olympic athletes. Broken line: length of the step in one of the athletes when running at a constant speed. The numbers on the right of the isopleths irradiating from the origin indicate the step frequency: this is about constant when running in acceleration: when running at a constant speed it is constant up to a speed of about 6 m s^{-1} (22 km h^{-1}) after which it increases with increasing speed. (From Cavagna *et al.* 1965.)

1963): this is presumably due to the greater braking component of this animal produced by its body architecture. This backward component will be greater the lower is the centre of gravity of the body and the longer the animal. In fact the angle α made by the force F exerted by the foot when this strikes the ground with the horizontal will be smaller, and the horizontal component $F \cos \alpha$, responsible for the braking action will be correspondingly greater. It may therefore be predicted that the greyhound would have a great advantage over the dachshund: I do not know whether comparative results of this type have ever been obtained.

Measurement of maximum muscular power during running

The measurement of maximum muscular power in man when running on the level is made difficult because of the rapid alternation of positive and negative work. This results in an underestimate for total work done. For this reason it has been stated erroneously that maximum muscular power cannot be exploited in running because the measured values are lower than those obtained for other types of exercise, such as rowing or cycling (in which practically no negative work is implied).

As mentioned above, the error due to the negative work component of this exercise may be eliminated by recording the potential energy of the body continuously, for example with a platform, so that positive and negative work are measured separately. Obviously the most practical method of measuring muscular power is to have a subject performing an exercise which involves only positive work: such as walking or running uphill at an incline higher than 20–30 per cent, or running in acceleration.

By measuring with the platform the potential energy of a man running at maximum acceleration a tracing such as that of Fig. 3.30 is obtained. It appears that in the first few steps the negative work is nil or inappreciable, all the work being positive and employed to increase the kinetic energy level of the subject: very soon, however, negative work (downward trend of the curve) at each step increases progressively to reach about the same value of the positive work when the average speed of the runner tends to a steady value.

The incline of the curve drawn through the maximum values of the oscillations of the graph of Fig. 3.30 is representative of the muscular power: it has a maximum value at zero time: the maximum muscular power. It decreases progressively as the amount of negative work performed at each step increases.

A similar graph, giving the changes in the potential and kinetic energy on the second and third step of a sprint at maximum acceleration in an Olympic runner is given in Fig. 3.31. In this athlete the maximum mechanical power during the first seconds was calculated to amount to $180 \, kg \, m \, s^{-1}$. This is of the same order of magnitude as the value obtained by Wilkie (1960) in other types of exercise (rowing, cycling) in which only positive work is performed.

Margaria and Coll (1966) have introduced a very simple method to measure the maximum anaerobic power in man. The subject runs up a staircase two steps at a time at maximum speed, and the vertical component of the speed of progression (see

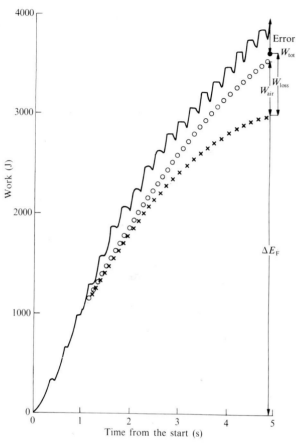

Fig. 3.30. The kinetic energy (J) necessary to move forward the centre of gravity of a man sprinting, as calculated from data obtained with a platform sensitive to horizontal forces only, as a function of the time from the start. The rise of the line indicates the positive work done, the horizontal tracks the 'flight' periods, and the decreasing parts the negative work. The continuous line indicates the work necessary to move the body forward, as calculated from the kinetic energy changes measured by the force exerted by the foot on the platform. The crosses indicate the kinetic energy of the body calculated from the actual speed in forward direction by measurement of the time taken to cover the distance between two photoelectric sights. By adding to this last value the work done against air resistance W_{air}, the curve indicated by open circles is obtained. The total work W_{tot} is the work actually done by the muscles to increase the kinetic energy E_F and to overcome friction against the air and within the body, W_{loss}. 'Error' is the difference between the kinetic energy actually gained by the runner and that calculated from the push of the foot on the ground. The difference between the curve indicated by the circles and the full line is possibly internal work plus work done against friction within the body to overcome anelastic deformation. (From Cavagna *et al.* 1971.)

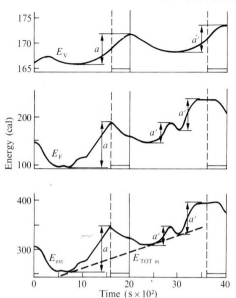

Fig. 3.31. Potential (upper curve), kinetic (middle), and total (lower) energy changes during the second and the third step from the start in sprint running at top speed in an Olympic athlete. *a* and *a'* indicate the positive work performed per step. The broken line gives the average total external energy changes of the body over this period. Abscissa: time-scale from beginning of second step: 0·01 s. (From Cavagna *et al.* 1965.)

p.   ) is measured with an electronic chronometer sensitive to 0·01 s.

For the same subject as in Fig. 3.31 a maximum vertical velocity of 2·8 m s^{-1}, corresponding to a power of 190 kg m s^{-1}, was recorded with this method—not appreciably different from that obtained with the much more complicated and time-consuming method of the platform.

The rate of positive and negative work in walking

Walking uphill, part of the increased potential energy acquired during the positive work phase of the step is not wasted, because the negative work in the following phase of the step is less than the positive. The negative work performed within a step cycle in fact decreases progressively with increasing gradient, and when walking at an incline of about 20 per cent it is no longer appreciable. The positive work per step, on the contrary, increases progressively with increasing steepness.

Walking downhill the opposite takes place: the lift of the body in the first half of the step becomes smaller with increasing gradient, becoming inappreciable at an incline of only about -10 per cent: for higher incline values the energy expenditure curve follows the $-1·2$ iso-efficiency line (see Fig. 3.10).

As the values for work given on the right-hand ordinate of Fig. 3.10 are in kilograms-metres per kilogram per metre, the same values are indicative of the pull, in kilograms per kilogram of body weight in the direction of the progression, needed to keep the body in motion at a constant average speed. This can be visualized as the equivalent constant pull necessary to meet the resistance to progression.

A constant pull of this amount would successfully replace the pull of the muscles, were this employed to meet either a frictional, or a gravitational resistance to progression. This however is not the case. In fact, considering that the equivalent pull involved walking on the level, corrected for the mechanical efficiency, amounts to 44 g per kilogram of body weight, and that when walking downhill on a 4·4 per cent incline the same pull is acting in the direction of the movement, one would expect the energy cost to be nil in the latter case. In reality the energy requirement is reduced; not to zero however, but to 60 per cent of the value for walking on the level; even on greater inclines the cost of walking is not reduced by less than 50 per cent.

That a constant pull cannot take over completely from the pull of the muscles is further evidence that the energy expended in walking on the level is not used to meet any resistance to progression, but to perform positive and negative work within the step cycle. This would certainly be the case for other kinds of locomotion, such as cycling, skating, swimming, etc., where only positive work is performed, and no negative work is involved in any phase of the exercise.

The muscular work done in walking or running could be replaced by an external pull only if positive (in the direction of the movement) and negative pulls were alternated in the appropriate phases of the step cycle. A constant positive pull, such as is exerted while walking downhill, can replace some or all the positive work performed by the muscles during a particular phase of the step cycle, but it will sum vectorially with the inertial forces during the negative work phase of the step. To save on muscular action in the negative work phase of the step, the pull would have to be reversed, i.e. directed backwards, and adjusted to the corresponding intensity. The intensity of the pull by the muscles, both the positive and the negative, is not constant, and therefore it would be very difficult to replace it by an external force (Margaria 1968).

The effect of a steady pull on the energy expenditure in walking

A schematic model of the effect and the efficiency of a constant external pull, when walking up or downhill, may be made by assuming that the positive work is performed during the first two-thirds and the negative work during the last third of the step cycle (see Fig. 3.15), and that both of them change at a constant rate, as indicated schematically in Fig. 3.32.

Assuming then that the pull forward, as it takes place in downhill walking, equals the pull of the positive work phase of the step, no positive work needs to be performed by the muscles in this interval: these will have to support only the negative work, which in the last third of the step phase will be higher than in walking on the level. This is what seems to take place at an incline of about -10 per cent, an incline value for which the experimental curve meets the $1 \cdot 2$ iso-efficiency line (Fig. 3.10).

Walking uphill the pull is in the direction opposite to progression, and only the negative work is supported. The experimental line meets the $0 \cdot 25$ iso-efficiency line at an incline of $+22$ per cent (Fig. 3.10), suggesting that about twice as great a pull than for positive work is necessary to take over the negative work when walking on the level. Assuming that when walking on an incline the positive and the negative work maintain the same intensity, and time-course characteristics as walking on the level, this seems to indicate that in walking on the level the negative pull is twice as great as, and lasts only half the time (or is carried for half the distance) of, the positive pull.

The fact that positive work performance lasts longer in the step cycle also explains the asymmetry of the curves of Fig. 3.27, i.e. the condition of minimum wasted work is reached at a lower incline in downhill than in uphill walking.

In effect, it appears from the work of Cavagna and others (Cavagna *et al.* 1963; Cavagna and Margaria 1966) that the energy expenditure takes place in two distinct phases of the step cycle, as indicated by *a* and *b* marked on the curve E_{ext} (Fig.

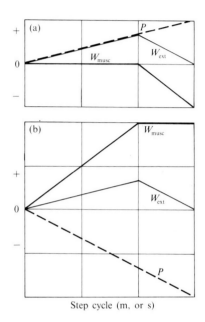

Step cycle (m. or s)

Fig. 3.32. Effect of a constant pull on the energy level of the body in a single step cycle. (a) Walking on the level with a steady applied positive pull such as *P*, leading to an energy change W_{ext}, equivalent to the energy change taking place during the positive work phase of the step. When walking normally without any pull, the work that must be accomplished by the muscles is $P - W_{ext} = W_{musc}$. (b) Still assuming that W_{ext} does not change when a negative pull is applied to the walking subject, such as when walking uphill, only positive work is performed by the muscles during the negative pull.

In (a) only negative work is performed; in (b) only positive work is performed. At incline values higher than +22 per cent or −9 per cent only one kind of work, either positive or negative, is performed and it can therefore easily be measured. (From Margaria 1968.)

3.13). These two phases of positive work are often smoothed in a single phase, and, except in the cases of walking at 4·92 km h⁻¹ and 6·31 km h⁻¹, no negative work is performed between the two, as shown in the curves of Fig. 3.15. Walking at a low speed positive work performance occurs over just about two-thirds of the cycle time, negative work being performed over the remaining third. At higher speed, the positive work phase is a progressively higher fraction of the cycle time, and the E_{ext} line corresponding to the negative work becomes very steep.

As shown in Fig. 3.15, positive and negative work actually performed do not follow such a smooth curve as in the schema of Fig. 3.32; and even if the average rate of positive work performance when walking on the level equals that due to the external pull, muscle activity is required when the increase of energy involved at a particular instant is higher than that due to the external steady pull: the same may be said about walking uphill, when a steady backward pull is active. In spite of this, however, the description above gives a sufficiently approximate quantitative explanation of the observed facts.

Similar arguments could be extended to running, only in this case the problem is complicated by the elastic energy accumulated and released by the muscles in certain phases of the step: utilization of the elastic energy can be made only by the muscles in the active state. On the other hand, as muscle activity requires energy expenditure in any case, a steady pull will never be able to reduce energy expenditure to zero in walking and running as is possible in other forms of progression such as freewheeling in cycling, skiing, swimming, etc.

The utilization of the elastic energy in muscular exercise

The observation that the elasticity of the muscle in contracted state has such an important role in muscular exercise that it accounts for about the half the positive work performed running on the level has been confirmed by many experiments in man and in an isolated frog muscle preparation.

Human subjects performed an exercise consisting of flexing the knees 15 times per minute in two different ways: in one case flexion and extension took place at regular intervals of 2 seconds each, and in the other extension followed the flexion immediately. In the first case the extensor muscles contracted in the downward movement to control the flexion, then they relaxed in the interval of 2 seconds before initiating the extension movement, i.e. that of positive work performance: the elastic energy stored during the negative work phase was therefore lost and transformed into heat. In contrast, in the case where extension followed flexion immediately, no relaxation took place between the negative and the positive work phases, and the elastic energy stored during the first phase could be utilized in the immediately following positive-work performance. The mechanical work performed was obviously the same in the two experiments, the number of flexions and extensions per minute being the same; oxygen consumption however was shown to be very appreciably less when the extension movement followed the flexion immediately; and the mechanical efficiency of this exercise was about 40 per cent greater. The subjects themselves found the

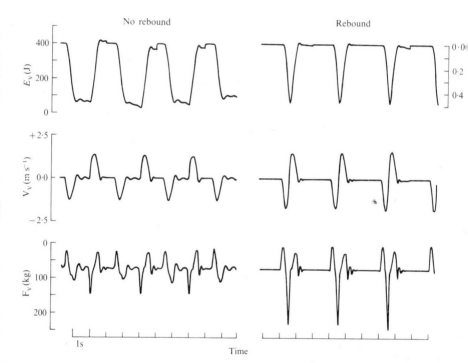

Fig. 3.33. Top tracing: Left ordinate, potential energy changes E_V, in joules; right ordinate, vertical displacement of the centre of gravity S_V, in meters. $S_V = 0$ indicates the position of the centre of gravity of the body in the erect position. v_V is the vertical speed of the centre of gravity in meters per second, as obtained by electronic integration from the bottom tracing. Bottom tracing: force exerted by the body on the platform (kg): subject weight is 71 kg. Tracings on the left refer to exercise performed with a pause between flexion and extension (no rebound); the tracings on the right, were obtained when extension immediately followed flexion (rebound). (From Thys *et al.* 1972.)

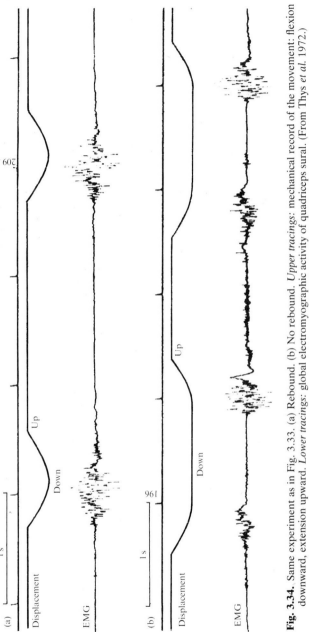

Fig. 3.34. Same experiment as in Fig. 3.33. (a) Rebound. (b) No rebound. *Upper tracings*: mechanical record of the movement: flexion downward, extension upward. *Lower tracings*: global electromyographic activity of quadriceps sural. (From Thys *et al.* 1972.)

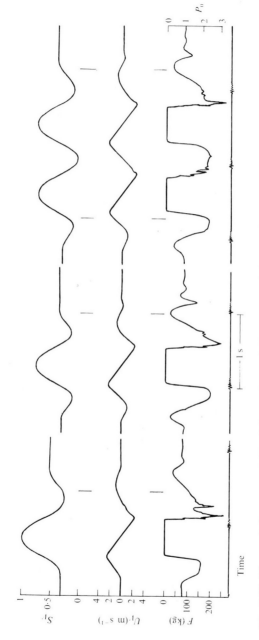

Fig. 3.35. The vertical component F_V of the resultant of all the external forces acting on the body (neglecting air resistance), the vertical velocity v_V and the vertical displacement s_V of the centre of gravity of the body are plotted as a function of time during a jump off both feet from a vertical force-sensitive platform. Right hand ordinate graduated in multiples of P_0, where P_0 is body weight. *Left:* the jump is performed starting with legs flexed. *Middle:* the jump is performed in the conventional way, the positive work performance being preceded by a rapid flexion of the knees ('bouncing') as indicated by the first upper wave of the F_V trace and the concomitant down waves in the v_V and S_V traces. *Right:* two successive jumps are performed in succession in the conventional way. (From Cavagna *et al.* 1971.)

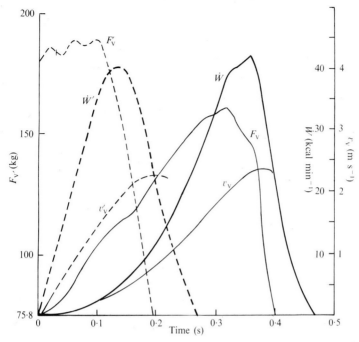

Fig. 3.36. Same experiment as in Fig. 3.35. Vertical force and velocity of the centre of gravity during most of the phase in which the previously stretched muscles (F'_V and v'_V; broken lines) and the unstretched muscles (F_V and v_V; continuous lines) perform positive work. The instaneous power $\dot{W} = Fv$ has also been calculated: this appears to be the same in both cases, but the time necessary to reach the maximum value is much shorter in the case where the extensor muscles have been previously stretched (W'): consequently the average power, calculated over the full time of positive work performance, appears to be much higher in the case of the previously stretched muscle. (From Cavagna *et al.* 1971.)

work performed by the second method much easier and less fatiguing (see Figs 3.33 and 3.34).

It is common experience that when performing a high jump the exercise is made much more difficult if started directly from being stationary in a flexed limbs position: we always start a vertical jump upright then spontaneously flex on the knees to stretch the extensor muscles of the limbs, which become 'loaded' with elastic energy. This mechanism is not, however, limited to jumping and knee-flexion exercises, but is a very general phenomenon: in nearly all exercises a contraction of the muscle in performing positive muscular work is preceded by the stretching of the muscle itself by gravitational or kinetic (inertial) forces.

Experiments have been performed on vertical jumps on a platform sensitive to vertical forces, and the push on the ground, the speed of the centre of gravity of the body and the time-course of the exercise have been recorded (Figs 3.35 and 3.36). The result obtained is that when the jump is preceded by a flexion of the lower limbs the *force* exerted by the muscles during the phase of positive work is much greater than when the jump starts from a flexed-limbs position which is not preceded by stretching. The vertical component of the *speed* of the centre of gravity of the body at the take-off, as well as the *instantaneous power* developed, are about the same for either method: but the *average power* developed in the 'bouncing' jump is much higher, because the time of positive work, which lasts until the take-off, is much shorter.

Utilization of the elastic energy in the isolated muscle. Force-length diagrams

The capacity of the isolated muscle to accomplish a greater amount of positive work when this is preceded by stretching has been shown by measuring the work performed by a muscle which is stretched and allowed to shorten at a given controlled speed by means of a Levin–Wymann muscular lever.

From the data of these experiments it has been possible to construct the tension–length diagram of the muscle subjected or not to previous stretching (see Figs 3.37 and 3.38). In my opinion, the conventional tension–length diagram of a muscle, obtained from isometric contractions of the muscle at different rest lengths, has a very limited significance, as it does not take into account the previous recent history of the muscle, which conditions to a great extent the tension that the muscle is able to develop. In other words the initial length is not the only factor responsible for the tension that the muscle may develop as a result of its activity; its immediately preceding activity may also have a very appreciable effect. The amount of work performed is given on force–length diagrams by the area delimited by the curve and the coordinates.

Obviously the amount of work performed depends on the initial length of the muscle: by stimulating the muscle tetanically

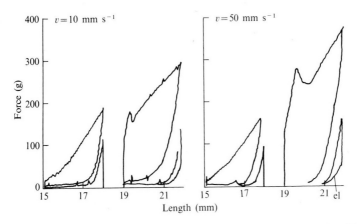

Fig. 3.37. Dynamic force–length diagram of an isolated frog gastrocnemius. The muscle, at an initial length of 18 mm or 21·8 mm was tetanically stimulated and then allowed to shorten at the speed v indicated. Alternatively, the muscle was tetanically stimulated when at a length of either 15 mm or 19 mm, stretched to the same length as before, i.e. 18 mm or 21·8 mm respectively and then allowed to shorten. The speed of stretching and of shortening were both the same, as indicated. The excess positive work due to stretching increased with muscle length and with speed of stretching.

The curve in the bottom right corner (el) is the force-length diagram of the parallel elastic elements, obtained during stretching the relaxed muscle. (From Cavagna *et al.* 1968.)

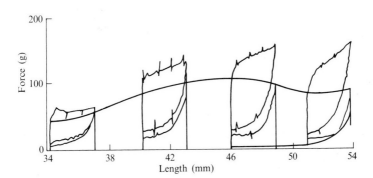

Fig. 3.38. Dynamic force–length diagram of a frog sartorius at four different initial lengths with and without previous stretching, as in the experiment of Fig. 3.37. A line was drawn through the maximum isometric tension values to obtain the conventional static force–length diagram. (From Cavagna *et al.* 1968.)

and then allowing it to shorten at a constant speed starting from the rest length of the muscle l_0, the work performed is less than when the muscle is stimulated at a lower length and then stretched to the length l_0 before it is allowed to shorten at the same speed. All other conditions being unchanged, a previous stretching of the muscle in contraction therefore appears appreciably to increase the work performance.

The area under the tension-length curve a+r of active muscle of Fig. 3.39 has been considered the *maximum potential work*. However, this concept has had to be modified, as the tension developed by the muscle in isometric contraction is not the maximum possible: a previously stretched muscle develops a much higher tension. Therefore the maximum potential work must be greater than that defined by the conventional tension–length diagram, by a variable amount which appears to be a function of the amplitude and speed of stretching.

These findings seem to have a great functional importance: in the past physiologists dealt substantially with only two types of

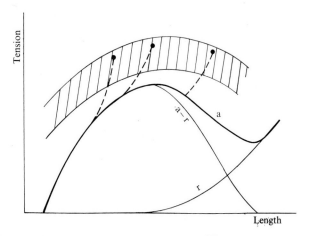

Fig. 3.39. Tension–length diagram of a muscle at rest (r) and in activity (a); isometric contraction. The curve a+r is the net result due to activity. The tension values due to stretching the contracted muscle (broken lines) fall approximately in the shaded area, depending on, among other factors, the initial length of the muscle and the speed of stretching.

The maximum potential work of the muscle is represented by the area between the a+r curve and the coordinates for the unstretched muscle. For previously stretched muscle this area would be appreciably greater.

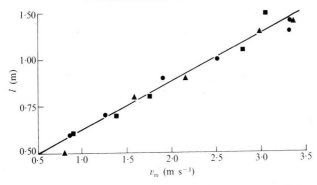

Fig. 3.40. Length of the steps as a function of the average walking speed. Different symbols indicate different subjects. (From Cavagna and Margaria 1966.)

contraction, *isotonic* and *isometric*. Isotonic contraction preceded by the stretching of the muscle has never been given much attention. This third type of contraction, however, is the most common type of muscular activity, met not only in running, in jumping, and in practically all sport movements, but also in all types of ordinary muscular activity. Purely isotonic or purely isometric contractions are exceptional.

Walking and running as oscillatory phenomena

It has been shown that in walking and running the length of the step l increases linearly with the average speed of progression (see Figs 3.29, 3.40, and 3.41). The isopleths radiating from zero in Fig. 3.29 indicate the *step frequency* per second, or its reciprocal value, the *duration of the step*.

For walking or running at a constant speed l does not start at zero: by extrapolating to zero the line drawn through the experimental data a value of about 0·3 m is obtained (Fig. 3.41).

The slope of the line is the time taken to cover the step length above 0·3 m: this time appears to be constant and independent of speed and step length, while the time employed to cover the other, constant, fraction of the step ($\sim 0\cdot3$ m) may change appreciably.

The fact that the time employed to cover l is a constant, being about 0·25–0·30 s, suggests that walking and running are phenomena of an oscillatory type, such as the swinging pendulum, for which the time of a full oscillation, i.e. the *period*, is

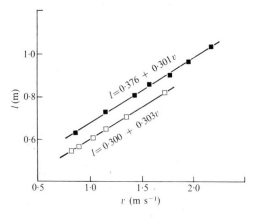

Fig. 3.41. Step length *l*, when walking on the level, as a function of speed of progression. *Upper:* subject G.M.; height 1·96 m; body weight 84 kg. *Lower:* subject G.P.; aged 15; height 1·47 m; body weight 42 kg. (From Margaria *et al.* 1966.)

also independent of the amplitude of the oscillation (the equivalent of the step length). The average linear speed of the oscillating mass of the pendulum corresponds to the average speed of progression of a man walking or running.

The main difference between walking or running and the movement of a pendulum is that in walking the oscillations take place in one direction only, thanks to the alternating action of the lower limbs. Another difference is that a relatively small fraction of the step length, equal to about the length of the foot, escapes this description.

The slope of the lines of Figs 3.29, 3.40, and 3.41 therefore have the significance of a period of oscillation of the body. Its value, about 0·3 s, corresponds to a step frequency of about 180–200 min^{-1}, which is just that which is found when running at 16–18 km h^{-1}.

About the same value for the frequency of oscillation of the body has been found by Cavagna (1970) on the damped oscillations of a subject at the end of a jump on a platform sensitive to vertical accelerations. It has been shown by Margaria *et al.* (1966) that the slope d*l*/d*v* of the line describing the step length as a function of the speed of progression always maintains the same value: whether the subject walks on the level or uphill or downhill; or when the body mass is increased by adding weights (by carrying a backsack of up to 40 kg). It has also been found to be the same for people of very different body sizes such as the two subjects of Fig. 3.41, the only difference being that the line for the shorter subject is displaced downward at a constant speed, so that the absolute value of the step frequency of the smaller subject is higher, due to a reduction, from 0·38 m to 0·30 m, of that fraction of the step length which is constant independent of speed of progression.

The period P of a simple pendulum is defined by the so-called 'law of the pendulum':

$$P = 2\pi\sqrt{\frac{L}{g}}$$

from which it appears that P depends only on the length L of the pendulum, and on the gravitational force g, being independent of the mass or the amplitude of the oscillations. A similar law may hold for man walking or running, thus supporting the opinion that this exercise is really of oscillatory or pendular type.

On this basis, it can be predicted that at reduced gravity, such as on the surface of the moon, the period of the system increases and the step frequency correspondingly decreases.

The linear increase of the step length as a function of the speed of progression is valid only for speed values not greater than 16–18 km h^{-1} when running at constant average speed. Speed higher than this value are essentially obtained at the expense of an increase of the step frequency while the step length tends to remain nearly constant (see Fig. 3.29). It could be argued that when running at high speed the limb muscles are contracted for a relatively longer time and that the tension they develop is greater, therefore giving the body as a whole a more rigid structure; consequently the period of oscillation of the system will decrease and the frequency will increase.

This hypothesis seems to be supported by the fact that when running in acceleration at low speeds, all the muscles are actively working to give to the body a very high forward acceleration. The step length is a linear function of the speed of progression for all speed ranges at low speed, but the period of oscillation in this case is small, although the speed is low, because the muscles are active. The period is about 0·2 s, corresponding to a step frequency of 250–300 or more per minute.

The influence of gravity on human locomotion

As described above (p.   ), when walking on the level at low speed the energy for the progression (kinetic) is mainly the result of the transformation of the potential energy stored in the first phase of the step when the body is lifted. The potential energy is given by

$$\dot{W}_V = PS_V = mgS_V,$$

where P is the body weight, m its mass, g the acceleration of gravity, and S_V the vertical displacement of the centre of gravity of the body.

On the moon surface, where the gravitation is one-sixth that on earth, the potential energy stored at each step will decrease (see Fig. 3.13). The gain of the kinetic energy into which this potential energy is transformed is therefore also decreased. This decrease of kinetic energy manifests itself as a reduction of the speed of progression: the speed of walking on the moon surface is not much higher than about 2 km h^{-1}.

This problem cannot be circumvented by increasing the potential energy. This goal could be achieved in two possible ways: the first by increasing the vertical displacement of the centre of gravity of the body S_V, but this is not possible as the lift of the body at each step is limited by the skeletal architecture of the lower limbs. (b) The potential energy could be increased by increasing the body mass m by adding weights. This does not in fact lead to an increase of speed even assuming that all the potential energy is transformed into kinetic energy. The kinetic energy should then be given by

$$\dot{W}_V = mgS_V = mv^2;$$

an increase of the mass m in the left-hand side of the equation involves an equal increase on the right-hand side: therefore v cannot be increased by increasing m. From the equation above it is evident that only by increasing g can an increase of the speed of progression be obtained.

The energy cost of locomotion in sub-gravity will be substantially reduced as less muscular activity will be required to produce the potential energy acquired in the first part of each step.

The step frequency will also be appreciably reduced on the lunar surface: in fact the falling forward of the body at each step, responsible for progression, takes place at a speed depending on the gravitational force: the time it takes for this falling is inversely proportional to the square root of the acceleration, and therefore the duration of the step will be increased in reduced gravity. The step frequency on the moon surface is only a fraction, $\sqrt{\frac{1}{6}} = 0{\cdot}4$, of the value observed on earth. Both the decreased body weight and the lower step frequency will lead to a lower energy expenditure when walking on the moon surface.

As previously stated, one substantial difference between walking and running is that in running the push of the foot on the ground is directed forward and upward: the potential and the kinetic components of the energy liberated increase simultaneously, and the transformation of potential energy into kinetic energy or vice versa is not possible. The potential energy acquired at each step in running must therefore be considered wasted, as it does not contribute to the displacement of the body in the direction of the progression (Margaria 1968). However, the vertical component of the push of the foot on the ground in running is necessary, because it is not possible to give a straight, forward push: the foot would slip on the ground. Furthermore a vertical lift of the body is necessary to displace the lower limbs during the very short time in which the body floats in the air and the feet have no contact with the ground: this time is very short because the vertical component of the push is just about equal to the gravitational force, independent of speed of running (Fig. 3.18).

The vertical component F_V of the total force exerted by the foot on the ground F can be defined as

$$F_V = mg + ma_V = P + F \sin \alpha$$

where $P = mg$ is the body weight, and $ma_V = F \sin \alpha$ the upward component of the push responsible for the upward acceleration, which, as stated above, is just about 1 g. The maximum value of the frontal component of the acceleration a_F in sprint running in compact soil has been found also to reach a value of about 1 g. The ratio of the vertical to the horizontal component of the total force exerted by the foot on the ground is therefore

$$\frac{mg + ma_V}{ma_F} = 2.$$

This is the value of the tangent of an angle of 63·5°. This is therefore the minimum angle necessary to prevent the foot slipping back in compact soil.

Running on ice or sandy soil where the coefficient of friction is less than for ordinary soil the push must necessarily be directed more vertically, and the forward component will be less. The frictional force F_f is in fact proportional to the vertical component of the total force exerted by the foot on the ground:

$$F_f = k(P + F \sin \alpha),$$

where the proportionality constant k is the *coefficient of friction:* for ordinary hard soil this is about 0·5.

Walking and running on the moon

If the vertical and the frontal components of the push are to equal the gravitational force on the moon, the speed of running cannot be higher than 12 km h^{-1}, provided that the soil is hard.

If the soil is slippery, as it is on the moon, where a thick layer of dust covers the surface of the ground, the coefficient of friction is reduced and the minimum angle made by the direction of the force impressed by the foot on the soil with the horizontal would have to be higher than 63·5°; the frontal component of this force would therefore be reduced, and the maximum speed of running would be correspondingly reduced to values not higher than $5–6 \text{ km h}^{-1}$.

Compensating mechanisms may take place in sub-gravity to

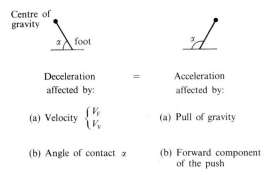

Deceleration   =   Acceleration
affected by: affected by:

(a) Velocity $\begin{cases} V_F \\ V_V \end{cases}$ (a) Pull of gravity

(b) Angle of contact α (b) Forward component
                                        of the push

Fig. 3.42. Schematic representation of the factors affecting the deceleration and the acceleration of the body at each step cycle when walking at a constant speed. (From Margaria *et al.* 1967.)

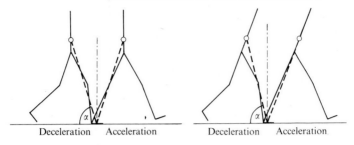

Fig. 3.43. Diagram showing a mechanism of compensation when walking in sub-gravity. By leaning forward, the angle of contact with the ground α is increased both during deceleration and acceleration. This decreases deceleration forward, and makes the action of gravity in accelerating the body forward more effective. (From Margaria *et al.* 1967.)

increase the speed of walking. For example (a) leaning forward so increasing the effective pull of gravity and decreasing the deceleration taking place when the foot strikes the ground; and (b) increasing the forward component of the push of the foot on the ground (Margaria, Cavagna, and Saiki 1967) (Figs 3.42 and 3.43).

As for running, an increase of the speed of progression cannot be achieved except by an increase in the leaning forward of the body, by which an increase of the forward component of the push of the foot on the ground can be obtained. This mechanism, however, has a limitation in the minimum value of the angle that the direction of the push makes with the horizontal, as described above (see Figs 3.44 and 3.45).

Running at constant speed:

Deceleration affected by:	=	Acceleration affected by:
(a) Speed of progression V_F		
		Forward component of the push
(b) Angle of contact α		

Fig. 3.44. Schematic representation of the factors affecting deceleration and acceleration at each step, when running at constant average speed.

Progressing by jumps in sub-gravity

An increased speed can be attained in sub-gravity by a substantial change of the mechanism of progression. Increasing the horizontal component of the push of the foot on the ground above the value critical for slipping can in fact be obtained only by correspondingly increasing the vertical component, so as to maintain the angle α above the minimal value. However, the vertical component of the push will then greatly exceed the acceleration of gravity so that the progression will have lost the

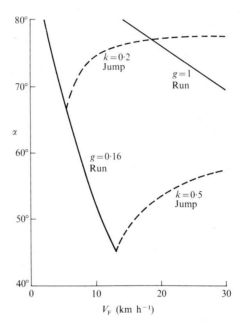

Fig. 3.45. The angle made by the direction of the dynamic component of the push of the foot on the ground with the horizontal at each step is plotted as a function of the mean speed of progression V_F. The line for $g = 1$ is constructed on experimental data, the line for $g = 0.16$ (surface of the moon) is calculated. At a speed of progression higher than that indicated by the origin of the broken lines on the line representing running on the moon, running, as conventionally defined, is no more possible, and progression takes place by jumping (broken line): the angle α then increases with speed.

The two broken lines have been calculated by assuming two different values of the coefficient of friction k for the lunar soil with the foot, as indicated. (From Margaria and Cavagna 1964.)

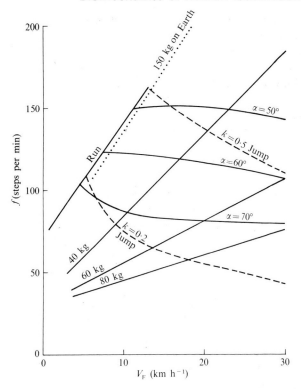

Fig. 3.46. Frequency of steps in running as a function of the speed of progression (full thick line); the same line also applies to moon surface conditions, up to the maximal speed of running as given by the origin of the broken lines (jumps). Step frequency in running increases with speed; in jumping it decreases with speed.

The iso-force lines are also drawn indicating the total mean force exerted by the foot on the moon surface at each step (straight thin full lines), and on the earth surface (single dotted line).

The iso-angle lines indicate the direction of the push of the foot, valid for $g = 0.16$. (From Margaria and Cavagna 1964.)

main *characteristic of running*, i.e. the component of the acceleration upward being equal to the gravitational force. A shift from *running* to a *jumping* mechanism will have taken place (see Fig. 3.45).

The duration of a single jump will be higher the larger the vertical component of the push; the step (or jump) frequency will be correspondingly lower. In Fig. 3.46 the step frequency (or the number of jumps per minute) is plotted as a function of the speed of progression. Iso-angle lines are shown for the values of the angle made by the horizontal with the direction of push of the foot on the ground from which the body weight component has been subtracted.

Energy cost of locomotion on the moon

The energy requirement for the progression at a given speed will certainly be much lower on the moon than on earth. In fact the energy required may be assumed proportional to the force exerted by the foot on the ground and to its time of application for each step. As the time involved in the push is essentially a function only of the speed of progression, it is easy to calculate from the data given in Fig. 3.46 that progressing at, say, 20 km h^{-1}, because of the lesser force exerted and the lower frequency of the jumps or steps, the energy expenditure per minute on the moon will be of the order of only one sixth that spent on earth.

The energy cost of progression per kilogram of body weight per kilometre covered on earth is about 1000 cal when running; this would be reduced to only 170 cal progressing by jumps on the moon at the same speed. This energy expenditure is not appreciably affected if (a) the jumps take place at a greater angle and are less frequent, as when the friction coefficient is small ($k = 0.2$), or (b) the jumps are more forwardly directed and have a higher frequency, for example where $k = 0.5$.

Only athletes can afford to maintain a speed of 20 km h^{-1} on earth, because of the high energy expenditure required—about $20 \text{ kcal per kg h}^{-1}$, equivalent to about 70 ml of oxygen per kilogram and per minute. Progressing at the same speed on the moon the oxygen requirement would be only about 11 ml per kg min^{-1}—less than walking on the level at 6 km h^{-1} on earth; practically everybody would be able to approach a speed of 50 km h^{-1} on the moon without becoming exhausted.

This conclusion is based on the assumption that the efficiency of running is the same on the moon as on earth. As mentioned above, the efficiency of running on earth, calculated conventionally, is very high, about 0.4–0.5, because of the utilization of the elastic energy stored in the muscles during the negative work phase of the step. It may be that on the moon, because of the different time-course of the stretching (negative work) and shortening (positive work) sequences of the muscles of the limbs, this utilization of the elastic energy stored in the muscles during the stretching phase is decreased, correspondingly increasing the energy expenditure.

The above discussion about the mechanics and energy cost of locomotion on the surface of the moon assumed that the freedom of movement of the subject is the same as on earth. According to the astronauts of Apollo 14 however, a space suit limits the extent of the movements by approximately 75 per cent, and, furthermore, the work required for movements of the same magnitude is greater. Unfortunately no data appear to be available of the energy cost of or of the mechanical work implied in the locomotion of a man wearing a space suit.

Because they have to wear space suits, the actual performance of astronauts running or jumping on the moon would be much poorer than calculated above.

Sprinting in sub-gravity

The forward acceleration of a good sprinter on earth at the start of a race may reach $10-15\ \mathrm{m\,s^{-2}}$ (Fig. 3.47); the step frequency may be of the order of $300\ \mathrm{min^{-1}}$ (see Fig. 3.29); the mechanical work per step amounts to 30 kg m. Such high values of forward

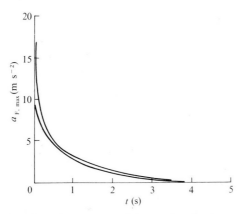

Fig. 3.47. Maximal frontal component of the acceleration in two athletes at the beginning of an all-out sprint. Same subjects as in Fig. 3.29. (From Cavagna *et al.* 1965.)

acceleration in sprinting cannot be reached on the moon, essentially because the step frequency cannot be as high as on earth: in fact a forward component of the push of the foot on the ground of the same order of magnitude as observed on earth would involve on the moon a very high vertical component of the push, and the body would be lifted by about 2 m: the time spent in the air would then be 3·1 s and the step frequency about $17 \, \text{min}^{-1}$.

The energy necessary to confer to the body a given forward speed v is $\frac{1}{2}mv^2$, and is independent of the gravitational force; it will therefore be the same on the moon as on earth; the work performed per unit time by the limb muscles will therefore be reduced on the moon roughly proportionally to the reduction of the step frequency. It can be calculated that on the moon at least 10 steps are necessary, over a time of at least 40 s, to reach the speed of $20 \, \text{km} \, \text{h}^{-1}$—a speed that a good sprinter on earth can reach in less than 2 s, performing the same number of steps. The maximum power developed when sprinting would therefore be reduced to about $\frac{1}{20}$ on the moon.

Sprinting on earth is an exercise that involves maximum muscular power: in the few seconds necessary to reach his maximum speed a good sprinter may spend an amount of energy equivalent to an oxygen consumption of $15 \, \text{l} \, \text{min}^{-1}$: on the moon no more than about $4 \, \text{kcal} \, \text{min}^{-1}$, or $0·8 \, \text{l} \, \text{min}^{-1}$ of oxygen are required.

The effect of gravity on jumping

As jumping is the most efficient method of progression on the surface of the moon, the biomechanics of this exercise at reduced gravity has been studied in detail: subjects have performed jumps from a platform sensitive to vertical acceleration both at normal and at simulated reduced gravity. Reduced gravity has been simulated by reducing the body weight of the subject by suspending him with long elastic ropes pulling on the shoulders, the trunk, and the inguinal region: the pull could be varied between 0 kg and 52 kg by regulating the tension of the elastic bands. The direction of the pull could be inverted to simulate increased gravitational force, as it occurs on planets heavier than earth, such as Jupiter, where $g = 2·7$ (Margaria and Cavagna 1971; Cavagna et al. 1972).

This method of simulating reduced or increased gravity is valid when the exercise consists of performing a vertical jump, as in these conditions the centre of gravity of the body remains on the line of traction of the elastic bands: it does not hold for simulating sub-gravity when walking or running, because in this exercise the centre of gravity of the body is displaced frontally or laterally within the body itself, as a consequence of the movements of the limbs, and the bands would generate a torque that would unbalance the body.

The experimental data obtained in simulated sub-gravity can be compared with those calculated on the assumption that the work performed in a maximal jump off both feet is the same at normal as at reduced gravity; the speed at the take-off, and the height of the jumps have been calculated for many values of g. It has been found that at 1 g in a subject weighing 66 kg the work performed in a maximal jump amounts to 51 kg m and the vertical velocity of the centre of gravity of the body at take-off amounts to $2 \cdot 6 \, \mathrm{m \, s^{-1}}$. This last parameter should increase at reduced gravity and decrease with increasing gravity, according to the function described by the curve of Fig. 3.48, the height of the jump changing correspondingly (ordinate at right of Fig. 3.48). The experiments made at simulated reduced gravity verify this: the recorded data fall significantly near the calculated curve. This is somewhat surprising, because in sub-gravity the resistance to the muscular action offered by the body weight is less: therefore the acceleration upward, and consequently the speed of shortening of the muscle, is increased. An increased speed of contraction may involve a change in the power developed, together with a reduction of the time of the positive-work performance.

The jumps were performed in two ways namely (a) starting from the erect position and flexing the legs (negative-work performance) immediately before giving the push (positive work), as occurs spontaneously when jumping (bouncing), or (b) starting the jump from the flexed-limbs position (no bouncing). The average power developed during the positive work phase in the bouncing exercise is maximal at 1 g, decreasing appreciably at lower and at higher gravitational force. When the jump is performed starting from flexed limbs, in the absence of bouncing, the power at 1 g is reduced by about 40 per cent: the power developed when jumping in this condition does not seem to be appreciably affected by the gravitational force (Fig. 3.49).

The effect of gravity on the push on the ground and on the

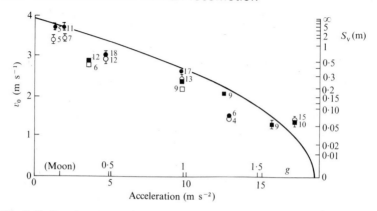

Fig. 3.48. Speed at the take-off V_0 in a standing jump off both feet as a function of gravity (abscissa: in m s^{-2} and in g units; M marks the Moon's gravity values). The continuous line has been calculated according to the equation $V_0 = \sqrt{\{2(W/m - gh)\}}$, where the mass of the subject $m = 66$ kg, the work $W = 51$ kg m, and the vertical height of the jump $h = 0.42$ m, as found on the earth. The ordinate on the right indicates the vertical lift of the centre of gravity above the take-off level, $S_V = v_0^2/2g$.

The experimental data (points out of the calculated curve) are the average of a number of jumps, as indicated; the standard error is also given when the bars exceed the size of the point. The full marks refer to the jumps preceded by stretching the contracted muscles, the open ones to the jumps without bounce (circles and squares two different subjects). (From Margaria and Cavagna 1972.)

vertical speed at take-off in maximal jumping from both feet is illustrated in Fig. 3.50, in which the force on the platform in jumping is plotted as a function of the vertical component of the speed of the centre of gravity of the body, both in the jumps with and without bouncing. The data are given for three simulated gravitational force levels: 1.8 g (dotted line); 1 g (continuous line); 0.2 g (dashed line). For each value of gravitation two curves start from the same point on the vertical line defining $v = 0$ and corresponding to the subject in the erect position on the platform immediately before performing the jump. The line directed diagonally upwards to the right corresponds to the jump without bouncing; the line directed downwards to the left to the jump with bouncing.

All the values to the left of the line defining $v_V = 0$ refer to *negative work*, namely the work done on the muscle; all the values to the right of that line refer to *positive work* performed by

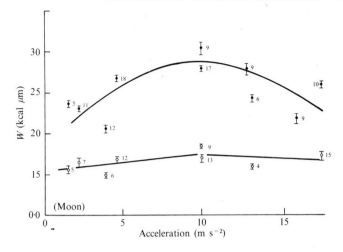

Fig. 3.49. Average power $\dot{W}$ developed per second in a maximal jump off both feet, plotted as a function of gravity. The two lines are traced by hand through the points: the upper one (full marks) refers to the jumps preceded by stretching the contracted muscles (bouncing), the lower one to the jumps from the flexed position (no bouncing). The difference between the two curves is maximal at 1 g and it decreases both at low and high g values. (From Margaria and Cavagna 1972.)

muscular activity. The areas under the individual curves and limited by the coordinates are indicative of the power.

It appears evident from this tracing that the difference between the bouncing and the no bouncing exercises is greatest at the beginning of the positive-work phase, the two curves tending thereafter to approach each other: this indicates that the maximum force is exerted by the muscles immediately after the stretching (see also Fig. 3.36) and also indicates the characteristic *transience* of the greater tension which results from the stretching.

The maximum vertical velocity of the centre of gravity of the body is only a little greater in the bouncing jump. One must remember that the time necessary to reach the maximum vertical velocity is much greater in the no bouncing jump, as described earlier (p. 119), because of the greater time the muscle in activity takes to stretch the series elastic elements: these are stretched much more rapidly, and without waste of chemical energy, by the

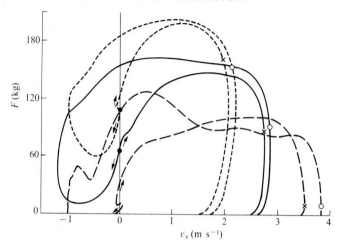

Fig. 3.50. Vertical component of the force F_V on the platform, as a function of the vertical component of the velocity of the centre of gravity v_V (negative values, downward movement; positive values, upward movement) in the 'bounce' and 'no bounce' jumps at different gravity values. Dotted line: 1·8 g; continuous line: 1·0 g; dashed line: 0·2 g. Two curves originate from each full point at $v_V = 0$, where the subject is in the erect position standing on the platform immediately before the jump: that going to the right corresponds to the jump without previous stretching, that going to the left refers to the jump preceded by stretching of the contracted muscles. The open points and the crosses on each tracing indicate the values of force and velocity developed when the centre of gravity is 12·6 cm below the take-off level. Assuming that at this instant the measured values of F_V and v_V differ from the actual force and speed of shortening of the muscles by the same factor, independently from g, the points and the crosses represent a part of the force–velocity curve of the muscles involved in the jump (including the length changes of the series elastic elements); as expected the force appears to be greater the smaller the speed.

weight of the body and by the inertial forces that act on the muscle in the phase of negative work.

It is this saving of chemical energy by the contractile elements of the muscle that gives the greater power and greater efficiency to the positive-work performance when the muscle has been previously stretched.

From Fig. 3.50 it appears also that the effect on greater tension and power developed in the phase of positive work due to stretching a contracted muscle is greater the greater is the stretching force, and the less is the extension and the time of the stretching.

The average power in a single 'bouncing' jump amount to about 200 kg m s^{-1} at 1 g, and it is reduced to about 160 kg m s^{-1} at the gravity of the moon. The height of a maximal jump on the moon will therefore be about 4 m, 4·4 s being spent in the air; this corresponds to a maximum frequency of the jumps of 12 min^{-1}.

As the work in a maximal jump is about 50 kg m, performing such jumps on the moon at a maximum frequency (12 min^{-1}) involves an amount of work of 600 kg m min^{-1}, or 1·35 kcal min^{-1}; and assuming a mechanical efficiency of 0·25 the energy expenditure will amount to about 5·5 kcal min^{-1}. This is well below the maximum aerobic pwoer of the subject—less than 50 per cent—so that it may be possible to progress on the moon by jumping on both feet, the mechanism kangaroos use on Earth.

This does not seem to have any advantage over progressing by alternate jumps on one foot only, which appears to be even more economical. In the last Apollo excursion on the moon, however, astronauts adopted the *jumping on both feet* method of locomotion, by which a reasonably high speed of progression, similar to fast walking on earth, could be reached: of course the height of the jumps was not very high, only a few centimetres, and the frequency of the jumps only about 50 min^{-1}, because of the mechanical limitations due to their space suits and to the fact that there was no necessity for them to travel any faster. The astronauts apparently carried out this exercise fairly effortlessly: a similar exercise on earth could certainly not be continued for even a limited time without resulting in exhaustion, particularly if the subject were handicapped by a space suit.

References

ABBOTT, B. C., AUBERT X. M., and HILL, A. V. (1951). The absorption of work by a muscle stretched during a single twitch or a short tetanus. *Proc. R. Soc.* B **139**, 86–117.

AGOSTONI, E., A. TAGLIETTI, and FERRARIO AGOSTONI, A. (1958). Composizione dell'aria alveolare e spazio morto respiratorio a diversi livelli metabolici. *Arch. Fisiol.* **58**, 1–14.

AMBROSOLI, G. and CERRETELLI P. (1970). Il rendimento della resintesi dei fosfati altamente energetici (ATP+CP) nel corso del ristoro anaerobico. *Boll. Soc. Biol. Sper.* **46**, 667–8.

ASMUSSEN, E. (1957). Determination of maximum working capacity at different ages in work with the legs or with the arms. *Scand. J. Clin. Lab. Inves.* **10**, 67–71.

ÅSTRAND, P. O., CLIDDY, T. E., SALTIN, B., and STENBERG, J. (1964). Cardiac output during submaximal and maximal work. *J. appl. Physiol.* **19**, 268–74.

—— and RHYMING, I. (1954). A nomogram for calculation of aerobic capacity (physical fitness) from pulse rate during submaximal work. *J. appl. Physiol.* **7**, 218–21.

BERGSTRÖM, J. (1967). Local changes of ATP and phosphorylcreatine in human muscle tissue in connection with exercise. *Circulation Res.* **20–21**, suppl. I, 91–6.

BRAMBILLA, I. and CERRETELLI, P. (1958). Determinazione del massimo consumo di ossigeno nel lavoro muscolare. *Boll. Soc. Biol. sper.* **34**, 678–9.

CAVAGNA, G. (1969). Travail méchanique dans la marche et la course. *J. Physiol., Paris*, suppl., **61**, 3–42.

—— (1970). Elastic bounce of the body. *J. appl. Physiol.* **29**, 279–82.

——, KOMAREK, L., CITTERIO, G., and MARGARIA, R. (1971). Power output of the previously stretched muscle. *Med. Sport* **6**, 159–67.

——, ——, and MAZZOLENI, S. (1971). The mechanics of sprint running. *J. Physiol., Lond.* **217**, 709–21.

——and MARGARIA, R. (1966). Mechanics of walking. *J. appl. Physiol.* **21**, 271–8.

——, ——, and ARCELLI, E. (1965). A high-speed motion picture analysis of the work performed in sprint running. *Encycl. Cinemat.* **5**, 310–19.

——, SAIBENE, F. P. and MARGARIA, R. (1963). External work in walking. *J. appl. Physiol.* **18**, 1–9.

——, ——, and MARGARIA, R. (1964). Mechanical work in running. *J. appl. Physiol.* **19**, 249–56.

——, ZAMBONI, A., FARAGGIANA, T., and MARGARIA, R. (1972). Jumping on the moon: power output at different gravity values. *Aerospace Med.* **43**, 408–14.

CERRETELLI, P. (1961). *Osservazioni fisiologiche, cliniche e psicologiche sul "Kanjut Sar" by G. Monzino*, Martelli publ., Milano.

—— and DEBIJADJI, R. (1964). The physiological effects of high altitude. pp. 242–47, Pergamon Press, Oxford.

——, di PRAMPERO, P. E. PIIPER, J. (1963) Energy balance of anaerobic work in the dog gastrocnemius muscle. *Am. J. Physiol.* **217,** 581–5.

——, PIIPER, J., MANGILI, F., RICCI, B., and CUTTICA, F. (1963). Il costo energetico della corsa nei cani. *Boll. Soc. Biol. sper.* **39,** 1806.

DAVIES, C. T. M. and BARNES, C. (1972). Negative (eccentric) work. Physiological responses to walking uphill and downhill on a motor-driven treadmill. *Ergonomics* **15,** 121–31.

——, SARGENT, A. J. and SMITH, B. (1974). The physiological response to running downhill. *Int. Z. angew. Physiol.* **32,** 187–94.

di PRAMPERO, P. E., PEETERS, L., and MARGARIA, R. (1973). Alactic O_2 debt and lactic acid production after exhausting exercise in man. *J. appl. Physiol.* **34,** 628–32.

——, and MARGARIA, R. (1968). Relationship between O_2 consumption, high energy phosphates and the kinetics of the O_2 debt in exercise. *Pflügers Arch. ges. Physiol.* **304,** 11–19.

—— and MARGARIA, R. (1969). Mechanical efficiency of phosphagen (ATP+CP) splitting and its speed of resynthesis. *Pflügers Arch. ges. Physiol.* **308,** 197–202.

DU BOIS-REYMOND, R. (1925). Der Luftwidentand des menschliches körpers. *Pflügers Arch. ges. Physiol.* **208,** 445.

EDWARDS, R. H. T., EKCLUND, L. G., HARRIS, R. C., HESSER, C. M., HULTMAN, E., MELCHER, A., and WIGERTZ, O. (1973). Cardiorespiratory and metabolic costs of continuous and intermittent exercise in man. *J. Physiol., Lond.* **234,** 481–97.

ELFTMAN, H. (1944). Skeletal and muscular systems: structure and function. *Medical physics*, pp. 1420–30. Year Book Publications, Chicago.

—— (1966). Biomechanics of muscle with particular application to studies of gait. *J. Bone Jt Surg.* **48–A,** 363–77.

EMBDEN, G. (1925). Säurebildung und energielieferung bei der muskelkontrakturen. *Ber. ges. Physiol. exp. Pharm.* **32,** 690–1.

FENN, W. O. (1930a). Frictional and kinetic factors in the work of sprint running. *Am. J. Physiol.* **92,** 583–611.

—— (1930b). Work against gravity and work due to velocity changes in running. *Am. J. Physiol.* **93,** 433–62.

—— (1957). Some elasticity problems in the human body. In *Tissue elasticity*, pp. 98–101, Remington, Washington, D.C.

—— and MARSH, B. S. (1935). Muscular force at different speeds of shortening. *J. Physiol., Lond.* **85,** 277–97.

HERMANSEN, L. and SALTIN, B. (1967). Blood lactate concentration during exercise at acute exposure to altitude. In *Exercise at altitude* (ed. R. Margaria), pp. 48–53. Excerpta Medica, Amsterdam.

HILL, A. V. (1927a). *Muscular movements in man: the factors governing speed and recovery from fatigue*, pp. 27–66. McGraw Hill, New York.

142 References

HILL, A. V. (1927b). The air resistance to a runner. *Proc. R. Soc. B* **102**, 380.

—— (1932). A revolution in muscle physiology. *Physiol. Rev.* **12**, 56–67.

—— (1938). The heat of shortening and the dynamics constants of muscle. *Proc. R. Soc. B* **126**, 136–95.

HULTMAN, E., BERGSTRÖM, J., and MCLENNAN ANDERSEN, N. (1967). Breakdown and resynthesis of phosphorylcreatine and adenosinetriphosphate in connection with immediate work in man. *Scand. J. clin. Lab. Invest.* **19**, 56–66.

JONES, D. A. (1973). Combined technique for studying the physiology and biochemistry of fatigue in the isolated soleus of the mouse. *J. Physiol., Lond.* **231**, 68P–69P.

KARLSSON J. (1971). Lactate and phosphagen concentration in working muscle of man. *Acta Physiol. scand.* Suppl., **358**, 7–72.

LAZAROVICI, V., MOLDOVAN, L., POPESCU, A., NUCZ, F., VRACIN, D., and SAC, A. (1970). L'influence de la température ambient sur la capacité d'effort physique des mineurs occupés à l'extraction des métaux non ferreux. *Ergonomics and physical environmental factors*, pp. 352 and 357. International Labour Office, Geneva.

LLOYD B. B. (1966). The energetics of running: an analysis of world records. *Adv. Sci.* **22**, 515.

LOHMANN, K. (1934). Über des chemismus der muskelkontraktion. *Naturwissenschaften* **22**, 409.

LUNDSGAARD, E. (1930). Untersuchungen über muskelkontraktionen ohne Milchsäurebildung. *Biochem. Z.* **217**, 167–77.

MARÉCHAL, G. (1964). *Le métabolisme de la phosphorilcréatine et de l'adénosintriphosphate durant la contraction musculaire*. Arscia, Bruxelles.

MARGARIA, R. (1938). Sulla fisiologia e specialmente sul consumo energetico della marcia e della corsa a varie velocità ed inclinazioni del terreno. *Atti Accad. Naz. Lincei Memorie*, serie VI, **7**, 299–368.

—— (1965). Una rappresentazione concisa di alcuni fondamentali dati funzionali respiratori e circolatori. *Arch. Fisiol.* **64**, 45–58.

—— (1967). Aerobic and anaerobic exercise. In *Exercise at altitude* (ed. R. Margaria), pp. 15–32. Excerpta Medica, Amsterdam.

—— (1968a). Positive and negative work performances and their efficiencies in human locomotion. *Int. Z. angew. Physiol.* **25**, 339–51.

—— (1968b). Capacity and power of the energy processes in muscular activity: their practical relevance in athletics. *Z. angew. Physiol.* **25**, 352–60.

—— (1972). Energy sources in muscular exercise. *Atti Accad. naz. Lincei Rc.*, Quaderno No. 178, 27–43.

——, AGHEMO, P., and ROVELLI, E. (1966a). Measurement of muscular power (anaerobic) in man. *J. appl. Physiol.* **21**, 1662–4.

——, ——, and —— (1966b). Determinazione nell'uomo della massima potenza musculare (anaerobica). *Atti Accad. naz. Lincei*, serie VIII, **40**, 23–8.

MARGARIA, R., AGHEMO, P., and SASSI, G. (1971). Lactic acid production in supramaximal exercise. *Pflügers. Arch. ges. Physiol.* **326**, 152–161.

——, CAMPORESI, E., AGHEMO, P., and SASSI, G. (1972). The effect of O_2 breathing on maximal aerobic power. *Pflügers Arch. ges. Physiol.* **336**, 225–35.

—— and CAVAGNA, G. (1964). Human locomotion in subgravity. *Aerospace Med.* **35**, 1140–6.

—— and —— (1971). Biomechanics of exercise at reduced gravity. *Proceedings of the 4th 'Man in space' Symposium*, Erevan, USSR. (In press.)

——, ——, and SAIKI, H. (1967). Human locomotion at reduced gravity. In *Life Science Research and Lunar Medicine, Proceedings of the 2nd Lunar Internal Laboratory Symposium*. Pergamon Press, Oxford.

——, CERRETELLI, P., AGHEMO, P., and SASSI, G. (1963a). Energy cost of running. *J. appl. Physiol.* **18**, 367–70.

——, ——, di PRAMPERO, P. E., MASSARI, C., and TORELLI, G. (1963b). Kinetics and mechanism of oxygen debt contraction in man. *J. appl. Physiol.* **18**, 371–7.

——, ——, and MANGILI, F. (1964). Balance and kinetics of anaerobic energy release during strenuous exercise in man. *J. appl. Physiol.* **19**, 623–8.

——, di PRAMPERO, P. E., AGHEMO, P., DEREVENCO, P., and MARIANI, M. (1971). Effect of a steady state exercise on maximal anaerobic power in man. *J. appl. Physiol.* **30**, 885–9.

—— and EDWARDS, H. T. (1934). The source of energy in muscular work performed in aerobic conditions. *Am. J. Physiol.* **108**, 341–8.

——, ——, and DILL, D. B. (1933). The possible mechanism of contracting and paying the oxygen debt and the role of lactic acid in muscular contraction. *Am. J. Physiol.* **106**, 689–715.

——, MANGILI, F., CUTTICA, F., and CERRETELLI, P. (1965). The kinetics of the oxygen consumption at the onset of muscular exercise in man. *Ergonomics* **8**, 49–54.

——, MILIC-EMILI, G., PETIT, J. M., and CAVAGNA, G. (1960). Mechanical work of breathing during muscular exercise. *J. appl. Physiol.* **15**, 354–8.

—— and MORUZZI, G. (1937). Il ristoro anaerobico del muscolo. *Arch. Fisiol.* **37**, 203–16.

——, OLIVA, R. D., di PRAMPERO, P. E., and CERRETELLI, P. (1969). Energy utilization in intermittent exercise of supramaximal intensity. *J. appl. Physiol.* **26**, 752–6.

MEYERHOF, O. (1930). *Die chemische Vorgänge in Muskel*. Springer, Berlin.

MILIC-EMILI, J. and PETIT, J. M. (1960). Mechanical efficiency of breathing. *J. appl. Physiol.* **15**, 359–62.

PIIPER, J., di PRAMPERO, P. E., CERRETELLI, P. (1968). Oxygen debt and high energy phosphates in grastrocnemius muscle of the dog. *Am. J. Physiol.* **215**, 523–31.

PUGH, L. G. C. E., GILL, M. B., LAHIRI, S., MILLEDGE, J. S., WARD, H. ,P., and WEST, J. B. (1964). Muscular exercise at great altitude. *J. app. Physiol.* **19,** 431–40.

ROVELLI, E. and AGHEMO, P. (1963). Physiological characteristics of the step exercise. *Int. Z. angew. Physiol.* **20,** 190–194.

ROWELL, L. B., BLACKMAN, J. R., MARTIN, R. H., MAZZARELLA, J. A., and BRUCE, R. A. (1965). Hepatic clearance of indocyanine green in man under thermal and exercise stresses. *J. appl. Physiol.* **20,** 384, 394.

SAIKI, H., MARGARIA, R., and CUTTICA, F. (1967). Lactic acid production in submaximal exercise. In *Exercise at altitude* (ed. R. Margaria), pp. 54–7. Excerpta Medica, Amsterdam.

SALTIN, S. and HERMANSEN, L. (1967). Glycogen stores and prolonged severe exercise. In *Nutritional and physical activity* (ed. G. Blix), p. 32. Almqvist & Wiksell, Uppsala.

SARGENT, R. M. (1926). The relation between oxygen requirement and speed in running. *Proc. R. Soc. B* **100,** 10–22.

STEGEMANN, J. (1963). *Forsch Ber. Landes NRhein-Westf.* n. 1178.

THYS, H., FARAGGIANA, T., and MARGARIA, R. (1972). Utilization of muscle elasticity in exercise. *J. appl. Physiol.* **32,** 491–4.

WILKIE, D. R. (1950). The relation between force and velocity in human muscle. *J. Physiol., Lond.* **110,** 249–80.

——. (1960). Man as a source of mechanical power. *Ergonomics* **3,** 1.

——. (1968). Heat work and phosphorylcreatine break-down in muscle. *J. Physiol., Lond.* **195,** 157–83.

Index

accelerometer, 81
adenosindiphosphate, 5
adenosintriphosphate, 5
alactic mechanism, 21, 23
altitude, effect of, 63
anaerobic reactions, 2
anoxia, 14, 60
alveolar air, 65
ATP, *see* adenosine triphosphate

blood, oxygen saturation, 60

carbon dioxide pressure in the alveoli, 65
cardiac output, 60
cycling, 112, 115
conversion engine, 1
CP, *see* creatine phosphate
creatine phosphate, 2

efficiency mechanical in locomotion, 74, 76
energetic processes in muscle hydraulic model, 53
energy from oxidations, 9
exercise,
    mechanical efficiency of, 55, 56
    intermittent, 46
    maximal, limiting factors, 65
    supramaximal, 9
exergonic processes in muscle, time course of, 23

friction coefficient in walking and running, 128

glycogen
    in muscle, 35
    resynthesis from lactic acid, 10
glycolysis, 2, 7
glycolitic mechanism, capacity and power, 20
GP, *see* phosphagen
gravity,
    effect on height of vertical jumps, 138
    effect of on human locomotion, 126
    effect on step frequency, 125

haemoglobin, 60
heart, minute-volume of, 60
heart rate, 60, 62
heart, stroke volume, 60, 62
high altitude, 60
Hill–Meyerhof theory, 2

jumping, effect of gravity on, 92, 134
jumps, progression by, 130

lactic acid,
    combustion coefficient, 5
    delayed formation, 27, 48
    diffusion, 10
    energy equivalent, 9, 13, 15; with phosphagen, 56
    in exercise, 12
    kinetics of, 4
    partition coefficient between water and fat, 17
    production in isolated muscle, 56
    in submaximal exercise, 18
    triggering mechanism for the production of, 26, 52, 58
locomotion, equivalent pull in, 112, 113
    mechanical model of, 105

monoiodoacetic acid, 2
Moon, locomotion on, 127, 128, 132, 139
muscle
    chemical reactions in, 6
    elastic energy in, 99
    elasticity, 115, 120
    as an engine, 1
    force–velocity diagram, 78
    isotonic and isometric contractions, 123
    maximum potential work, 122
    tension–length diagram, 122
    viscosity, 67, 73, 80, 100
muscular power, aerobic and anaerobic, 34, 35
    aerobic, measurement, 37; and performance in running, 43
    maximal, 21; measurement, 35
    in running, 108

old age, 63
oxidations, 7
oxidation potential in muscle, 26, 27
oxygen breathing, 60
  in exercise, 13, 14
oxygen
  consumption, in exercise, 12
    maximum, 10; in anoxia, 14
  debt, 3, 29
    alactic, 5, 24, 25, 29, 31; max-
      imum, 25
    lactacid, 5
    in maximal and supramaximal ex-
      ercise, 50
    net and gross, 32
    payment, 30; kinetics of, 4, 26; in
      strenuous exercise, 25
    time for contraction, and payment,
      34, 50
  energy equivalent of, 8, 9
  limit to maximal consumption, 14
  pulse, 62
  stores in the body, 32

pendulum, law of the, 125
phosphagen, 7
  cleavage in isolated muscle, 56
  content in muscle, 23
  efficiency of resynthesis, 55
  energy equivalent of, 23
  resynthesis, velocity constant of, 31
power, 9
  anaerobic, measurement of, 35
  maximum aerobic, 17, 21, 23

recovery, anaerobic, 27
resistance in walking and running, 100

running,
  energy cost of, 73
  mechanics of, 89
  mechanical model of, 94
  speed, relation to muscular power,
    44
  step frequency in, 107, 124

skating, 112, 115
sprinting, energy in, 133
steady state, 9
step length as function of speed in
  walking, 123
stepping exercise, energy cost of, 39
stroboscope, 81
swimming, 112, 115

treadmill, 68

ventilation, alveolar, 65
ventilation–perfusion ratio, 65

walking,
  energy cost of, 67
  high speed, 87
  mechanical model of, 85
  work in, 84; positive and negative,
    111
wind effect in locomotion, 101
work,
  external and internal, 83
  measurement of, in walking, 81
  negative, 75
  positive and negative, 77
  submaximal, 9
  wasted in locomotion, 103